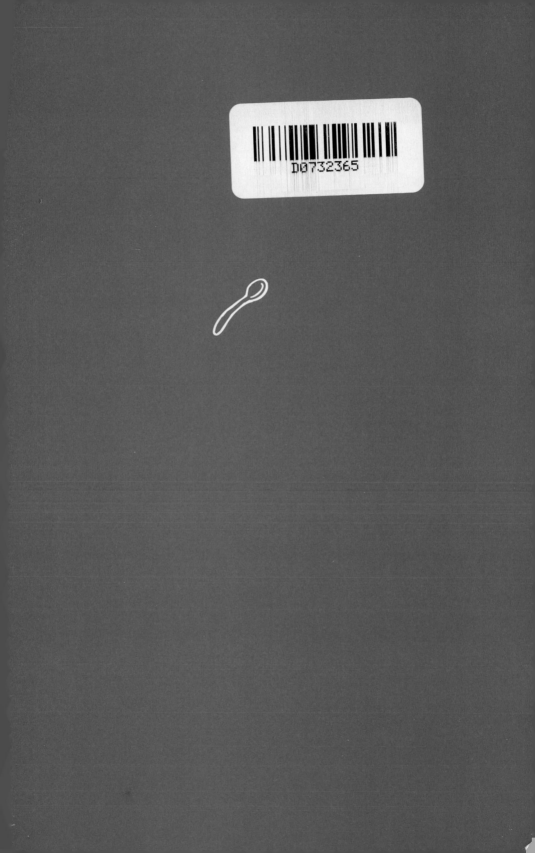

BRENDA BRADSHAW &
LAUREN DONALDSON BRAMLEY, M.D.

the Baby's

OVER 100 EASY, HEALTHY AND HOMEMADE RECIPES FOR

THE PICKIEST, MOST DESERVING EATERS ON THE PLANET

Table

RANDOM HOUSE CANADA

www.randomhouse.ca

Random House Canada and colophon are trademarks

NATIONAL LIBRARY OF CANADA CATALOGUING IN PUBLICATION

Bradshaw, Brenda (Brenda E.)
The baby's table : over 100 easy, healthy and homemade recipes for
the pickiest, most deserving eaters on the planet / Brenda Bradshaw and
Lauren Donaldson Bramley.

Includes bibliographical references and index.

ISBN-13: 978-0-679-31291-8
ISBN-10: 0-679-31291-9

1. Cookery (Baby foods)   2. Infants—Nutrition.
I. Bramley, Lauren Donaldson   II. Title.

RJ216.B663 2004   641.5'622   C2003-906888-9

Design by CS Richardson

Front cover photographs clockwise from left:
Jules Frazier, Ken Usami, Photodisc, Barbara Penoyar (all Getty Images)

Printed and bound in Canada

10 9 8 7 6 5 4 3 2 1

To the babies who inspired us

The Baby's Table Contains:

Foreword

As a general consultant pediatrician, I've been fielding questions for years from new parents about what (and how) to feed their children. When I first started my practice, I am embarrassed to say, many of these questions truly stumped me: When can I stop warming up the bottle? When can I give the baby eggs? Juice? Yogurt? It wasn't until I had children of my own that I realized how much there truly is to learn about the care and feeding of babies. And, alas, knowing how and what to feed a baby and putting it into practice are two different things.

The Baby's Table is full of delicious ideas and recipes. While some of the recipes may sound intimidating to the sleep-deprived new parent (Gourmet Tuna Melts or Salmon and Vegetables with Creamy Dill Sauce), they are all surprisingly simple and quick to prepare. When Mom and Dad are craving their favorite spicy take-out, having some of the dishes frozen in bulk to feed baby is a great option.

This book—part recipe book, part everything-you-need-to-know-to-feed-a-baby—answers all the feeding and nutrition questions I tried to answer in my early years as a pediatrician as well as the questions I had when I was figuring it out for myself as a new parent. The dishes are truly great-tasting as well as nutritious and safe. They focus on unprocessed, unsweetened and unsalted whole foods.

Finally! A book that I will be happy to recommend to new parents, to help them feed their baby for those crucial first years.

Cheryl L. Mutch M.D., C.M., F.R.C.P(C.)
Pediatrician, Burnaby, B.C., Canada

Introduction

If you're like many new parents, you may find the prospect of making your own baby food a daunting one. You're no Naked Chef; baby's keeping you busy (and tired)— and besides, how would you know that what you're feeding your infant is safe and supplies the nutrients needed for healthy development?

It's easier than you think. And *The Baby's Table*, filled with important nutritional information and cooking tips and more than 100 simple and tasty recipes, can show you how. There are helpful hints on dealing with behavioral issues such as feeding problems, and strategies for making healthy eating a pleasurable experience—for you as well as for your baby.

More and more parents today are seeing the advantages of preparing homemade baby food. It's nutritional, economical and takes far less time than you think. All you need is a steamer basket, a blender or food processor, a small double-boiler, ice cube trays and a freezer. In an afternoon—during one of baby's naptimes—you can whip up and freeze an entire month's supply of meals rich in essential nutrients.

Your baby's nutrition is of critical importance for physical and intellectual growth and development and has lasting implications for his or her future. Using the tips, recipes and meal plans provided in *The Baby's Table,* you can create your own baby-pleasing fare that offers nutritional advantages not found in commercial brands. Homemade baby food cuts down on unwanted additives and offers your baby a wider variety of textures and flavors than commercial baby food could hope to replicate. The savings are substantial; your own baby food can be prepared at a fraction of the cost of store-bought. In the long term, offering home-prepared baby food can also help you shape your baby's food choices for a healthy childhood, and beyond.

All recipes in *The Baby's Table* have been reviewed by a physician and tested by parents—and more importantly, babies! Information is based on the latest medical and nutritional research and complies with the current Canadian guidelines for infant feeding. Be aware that the contents of this book are not intended as medical advice: the suggestions apply only to healthy full-term infants, and parents should consult with their doctor before undertaking any change in their infant's diet.

The chapters in *The Baby's Table* are conveniently named for the age group to which the recipes apply: Newborn to Six Months; From Six Months; From Seven Months; From Eight Months; and Toddlers. There are also three helpful Appendices: Resources, Growth Charts, and References. For the purposes of this cookbook, age definitions are as follows: *newborn,* up to one month; *infant,* from birth to 12 months; *toddler,* from 1 to 3 years; and *child,* 3 years and older.

The fact that you're reading this book shows you're ready to take the plunge. Congratulations—you have made a commitment to a healthy future for your baby. Read on, have fun, be creative— and, since you're sure to be taste-testing these recipes yourself, *bon appétit!*

Newborn to Six Months

For the first 6 months your baby will be fed only breast milk or breast milk substitute. The first 6 months is a time of peak growth and bonding, when your baby will double or triple his birth weight, will learn to smile and laugh and will rely on you entirely for healthy nutrition. It has been proven that breast milk is the optimum nutrition for young babies. It is not always possible to breastfeed, however. Regardless of whether it is breast or bottle, a loving and caring approach to feeding will ensure your baby thrives to her greatest potential.

BREASTFEEDING

According to the Canadian Paediatric Society, the Dietitians of Canada, Health Canada and The American Academy of Pediatrics, breastfeeding is the optimum method of feeding for all infants with very few exceptions. Research continues to prove the vast benefits of breastfeeding for your baby:

▶ *Reduced rates of infection:* Breastfeeding has been shown to reduce the rates of respiratory, ear, gastrointestinal, urinary tract and other infections in both infancy and childhood by at least 30 to 50 percent. Antibodies and other proteins from the mother prevent infection and strengthen the immune system.

▶ *Possible prevention of Sudden Infant Death Syndrome (SIDS):* In addition to placing an infant on his or her back for sleep, recent studies show a reduced risk of SIDS among breastfed infants.

▶ *Enhanced cognitive development:* Breastfeeding has been shown to improve childhood intelligence quotient (IQ), standardized tests of reading, mathematics and scholastic ability. These improvements are thought in part to be due to the specific fatty acids found only in breast milk.

▶ *Prevention of allergies:* Breast milk provides protection against the development of allergies in those infants with a family history.

▶ *Prevention of iron deficiency:* Breast milk is associated with lower rates of iron deficiency, provided iron-fortified cereals are not postponed much beyond 6 months.

▶ *Other benefits:* There is a possible reduction in asthma, diabetes, bowel diseases and some childhood cancers in breastfed children.

And then there are the health benefits of breastfeeding for mothers:

▶ *Decreased osteoporosis in later life:* During pregnancy, calcium is lost from the mother's bones as a source for the developing baby. The hormones produced by breastfeeding replace the skeletal calcium lost during pregnancy, which leads to a decrease in osteoporosis.

▶ *Decreased cancer risk:* Breastfeeding is associated with a reduced risk of ovarian and breast cancer. This is thought to be due to the reduced levels of estrogen caused by breastfeeding.

▶ *Enhanced weight loss:* Breastfeeding is related to increased weight loss following birth and a faster return to pre-pregnancy weight and body shape. This process begins immediately, as hormones released during breastfeeding promote faster shrinkage of the uterus and mobilization of fat from the lower body. These effects occur without dieting or excessive exercise and are more evident with prolonged breastfeeding.

▶ *Other benefits:* New parents are often overwhelmed by the time commitment of breastfeeding a newborn baby. However, breastfeeding is an excellent way to escape the demands of cleaning, sterilizing and preparing bottles, particularly in the early weeks of baby's life. Furthermore, breast milk is a dynamic substance, which alters its consistency depending on both climate and your baby's needs.

HOW LONG? Many benefits can be achieved with 6 months of exclusive breastfeeding. For this reason Health Canada recommends at least 6 months of exclusive breastfeeding followed by the introduction of iron-fortified solid foods. It is ideal to continue breastfeeding for the first two years and beyond, if possible, as many of the benefits are more marked with prolonged breastfeeding. However, should extended breastfeeding not be possible, the benefits of even a short time are evident.

Eat well and avoid calorie-restricted diets during breastfeeding to ensure adequate energy for milk production. The composition of breast milk will vary according to your diet. The fat-soluble vitamins A, D, E and K and minerals are drawn from storage in your body so that your recent dietary deficiencies are not evident in the breast milk. The water-soluble vitamins C and B-complex are not stored by you and may therefore be deficient in breast milk if you don't meet your dietary needs. Many women choose to continue taking their prenatal vitamin throughout breastfeeding. In some countries, DHA, a type of omega-3 fatty acid, is now included in prenatal vitamins to improve infant brain and eye development and ward off post-natal depression. Speak to your doctor about the possibility of taking a DHA supplement while breastfeeding. If you consume a strict vegetarian diet you will likely be advised by your doctor to take a daily vitamin supplement. All women should drink plenty of fluids while breastfeeding, as it is easy to become dehydrated, which may then lead to exhaustion.

HOW TO GET STARTED Ideally breastfeeding should begin as soon as possible after birth. For the first 48 to 72 hours, breast milk consists only of a clear substance called colostrum. Colostrum is extremely rich in antibodies and plays a crucial role in development of the infant's immune system. As colostrum is low in calories, the breastfed newborn will lose weight in the first 3 to 4 days of life. Early breastfeeding patterns can be very erratic, and parents may think the baby couldn't possibly be getting enough; however, the infant has a good reserve to help her withstand this early phase. Weight loss is a normal part of early life and it is important for parents not to be discouraged. It is also important to resist supplementing colostrum with formula, or "sugar water" as was once common practice in many hospitals. Today these measures are only taken if medically necessary and are not for normal weight loss alone. The best treatment for the "hungry" baby is more practice at breastfeeding. This also encourages the breast milk to replace colostrum within 2 to 4 days.

In the early weeks newborns should be breastfed whenever they show signs of hunger. Early signs of hunger include increased activity, opening the mouth and turning the head in search of food, or attempting to "latch on." Crying is a late sign of hunger. Once milk has replaced the colostrum, newborns will feed approximately eight to ten times in 24 hours. It is important to hold baby upright for burping following a feed; however, babies may occasionally not burp and need not be continuously patted to do so.

At 1 week of age, adequate breastfeeding is indicated by at least six wet diapers and three to four stools per day. In these early weeks newborns who have not nursed for a period of 4 hours should be roused to feed.

In time, the duration of each feed will become shorter and nursing will occur less frequently. Sometime after the first month, babies may be encouraged to have fewer feeds during night hours with increased duration of morning feeds. This may be accomplished by comforting the baby in other ways, such as holding, rocking or changing.

If discharged from the hospital less than 48 hours after delivery, babies should be evaluated by a health care professional within the first 5 days of life. You should contact your doctor about possible inadequate feeding, the appearance of a yellow tinge to the skin or whites of the eyes (jaundice), vomiting or temperature above 100.4°F/38.0°C.

For concerns regarding breastfeeding, contact your doctor, community nurse or local La Leche League.

VITAMIN SUPPLEMENTATION OF BREASTFED INFANTS Vitamin D is important for normal bone growth and prevention of rickets in children and osteoporosis in adults. It is produced naturally when skin is exposed to sunlight but not always in sufficient quantities. This may be due to decreased exposure to sunlight, use of sunscreen and absence of vitamin D–stimulating rays in northern latitudes during the winter months. To overcome these factors vitamin D has been added to milk, margarine and infant formula in some countries. As breastfed babies do not consume these, they may become deficient in vitamin D.

The Canadian Paediatric Society and The American Academy of Pediatrics have recommended that all breastfed infants in North America be given supplemental vitamin D from birth until they can reliably obtain vitamin D through formula-feeding or vitamin D–fortified milk. Vitamin D supplementation can be given in the form of drops directly to the infant's mouth. This is also recommended for babies in other countries with a northern latitude or limited sunlight, particularly in winter months. According to the most recent Health Canada recommendations, all healthy term infants should receive a Vitamin D supplement of 400 IU daily from birth until the infant's diet includes at least 400 IU from other sources or until the breastfed infant reaches one year of age. Consult your doctor for a recommended brand.

Many parents wonder about the use of iron supplements for breastfed babies. It is true that iron is present in low quantities in breast milk; however, this iron is easily absorbed by the infant and is adequate for the first 6 months of life. There are also iron stores accumulated in utero. At 6 months iron-fortified cereals should be introduced to offset the depleting iron stores. In pre-term infants and infants with a birth weight less than 5.5 pounds (2.5 kg) it will likely be necessary to provide an iron supplement before 6 months. Again, consult your doctor for a recommended brand and dose.

EXPRESSING AND STORING BREAST MILK Once breastfeeding is well established you can return to work and still provide expressed breast milk for your baby. By using a portable electric, manual or battery-operated breast pump, you can express during breaks and lunch hours. The breast milk can then be stored in sterilized containers in the refrigerator. Many women begin to express and freeze breast milk prior to their anticipated return to work. Breast milk can be stored in the freezer for up to 1 month and in the refrigerator for up to 24 hours. All equipment, storage containers and bottles must be sterilized. For further information contact your doctor, local community nurse or La Leche League.

PRECAUTIONS DURING BREASTFEEDING Certain groups of women may be advised not to breastfeed, including women with active tuberculosis, HIV or AIDS. If you suffer from one of these conditions, review with your doctor the use of any medication, including over-the-counter drugs and herbal remedies.

Nursing women are advised not to exceed minimal and infrequent alcohol consumption while breastfeeding. Alcohol appears in breast milk at similar levels to that in the mother's blood. Small amounts of alcohol render the baby's resultant blood alcohol level very low because of dilution by the baby's body water. Larger quantities, however, may result in harmful blood alcohol levels. Studies have shown impaired motor function of infants whose mothers consume at least 1 drink each day. Contrary to popular thought, alcohol in breast milk has been shown to decrease infant's sleep and increase wakings within the period following intake. Women who have consumed alcohol are advised to wait at least 1 hour per standard drink prior to breastfeeding to allow some clearance of alcohol from breast milk. Women should not use any illegal drugs of abuse such as marijuana, cocaine, heroin and amphetamines at any time while breastfeeding.

WARMING THE MILK

When warming bags or bottles of breast milk or infant formula, use warm running water, an electric bottle warmer, or the stovetop on low heat. Do not use a microwave, as pockets of overheated milk may exist even if the temperature feels fine on your wrist. Furthermore, studies have found that high heat can alter the composition of breast milk, most importantly, the anti-infective properties of antibodies. There is no need to warm bottles of breast milk or infant formula. On summer days your baby may prefer a chilled bottle.

Studies comparing the cognitive function in babies suggest that those who were breastfed have a developmental advantage and therefore improved cognitive function as measured by IQ tests over those who were formula-fed. This has been attributed in some studies to the long-chain poly-unsaturated fatty acids omega-3 and omega-6. Both of these fatty acids are present in breast milk in the form of DHA and AHA. As these fatty acids constitute the majority of the brain and retina it has been proposed that their presence in breast milk is the reason for observed differences in cognitive ability. DHA and AHA, also referred to as "Lipil," have now been synthesized and added to some infant formulas. These formulas have long been available in the U.K., Europe and Australia and more recently in Canada and the U.S. These formulas may have "Omega-3," "DHA/AHA" and "Lipil" listed in the ingredients.

FORMULA-FEEDING

Breast milk is the ideal source of nutrition for infants. However, when breastfeeding is not possible, infant formula is the best alternative. In recent years infant formula has been developed to such an extent that it is viewed as a nutritionally complete food source for infants under 6 months. Research on improving infant formula continues, particularly in the area of fatty acid supplementation.

Only formulas specifically labeled as infant formula should be given to babies less than 1 year of age. There are a number of different brands and preparations of infant formula, but the preparation used by the majority of infants should be iron-fortified formula based on cow's milk. The cow's milk protein used in infants' formula has been isolated and modified from whole cow's milk to a form that is tolerated by infants.

IRON-FORTIFIED COW'S MILK PROTEIN-BASED FORMULAS This is the standard breast milk substitute for healthy, term infants. Brands of formula may differ in whether they contain certain additional compounds equal to those found in breast milk. Compounds most recently added to certain brands of infant formulas are those derived from the omega-3 fatty acids. The names "DHA/AHA," "Omega-3" or "Lipil" indicate that omega-3 fatty acids have been added.

SOY PROTEIN-BASED FORMULAS Despite widespread use of soy formulas there are only three indications for its use: a rare metabolic disorder called galactosemia, lactase deficiency, and some vegetarian diets. Furthermore, recent studies suggest that the phytoestrogens (compounds that mimic female hormones) in soy formula may be problematic: they may be linked to adult cancers and may cause younger onset of puberty. The significance of these findings remains unclear and research continues. Using soy protein–based formula unnecessarily may pose certain health risks for your baby. Do not use soy protein–based formula without consulting your doctor.

WHAT IS TAURINE?

In an effort to reproduce the benefits of breast milk, taurine has recently been added to some brands of infant formula. This amino acid is found in high levels in the brain, heart and retina, where it performs many important functions. Most notably, taurine is involved in the chemical reactions essential for normal vision, and deficiencies of taurine can cause degradation of the retina. Taurine is found in meat, fish and breast milk and is now often added to infant formula.

LACTOSE-FREE COW'S MILK PROTEIN-BASED FORMULAS This formula is used for babies who have been diagnosed as lactose intolerant. Your doctor will confirm this diagnosis through laboratory tests.

PROTEIN HYDROSYLATE FORMULAS (HYPOALLERGENIC FORMULAS) These formulas are used only for babies who may be at risk of developing allergies or who have a confirmed allergy to cow's milk proteins or soy proteins. Do not use this formula without a doctor's advice.

FOLLOW-UP FORMULAS Follow-up formulas are designed to be used by infants in the second 6 months of life. Compared with cow's milk they contain more nutrients and are more readily absorbed fatty acids. Pasteurized whole cow's milk may be introduced at 12 months of age.

BOTTLE STERILIZATION Correct preparation, cleaning and sterilization of all bottles and storage containers for expressed breast milk and formula is critical for the safety of your baby. Bacteria can grow in breast milk or formula and may cause gastroenteritis. All equipment must be thoroughly cleaned and then sterilized either on the stovetop or with a microwave or electric sterilization unit. Sterilization should continue until at least 3 months of age for a healthy, full-term baby. At this time your baby's gastrointestinal system is able to kill the bacteria. Always ensure that water used for formula preparation has been boiled for at least 3 minutes.

WATER Water used to prepare infant formula or baby food, and water offered for drinking must be free of chemical and microbiological contamination.

▶ *Tap Water:* When using tap water, allow the tap to run freely for 2 minutes each morning to flush out contaminants such as lead and copper that may have accumulated overnight. Also, use only water from the cold water tap as hot water may leach more contaminants from pipes.
▶ *Commercially Bottled Non-carbonated Water:* Commercially bottled waters suitable for use by infants are natural spring water drawn from underground springs and treated water, both of which have low mineral content. Mineral water, treated water with a high mineral content, and carbonated water are not suitable as they may be difficult for the infant's kidneys to metabolize.

► *Home Water Filters:* Home water treatment can be used to filter tap water but may pose additional problems. Charcoal filters may be a source of bacterial or silver contamination, and some softeners may add excess sodium. To enquire about your home water treatment equipment, contact the Criteria Section, Bureau of Chemical Standards, Health Canada (see Appendix I).

FLUORIDE

Fluoridation of the water supply is the most effective way to prevent dental cavities. However, many parts of Canada and other countries do not have fluoridated water. Recommended levels of fluoride have trended downwards in the past 10 years in an effort to reduce the incidence of dental fluorosis. Dental fluorosis occurs as a result of excessive fluoride exposure. It is characterized by white streaks or specks or brown-gray staining of the teeth. The teeth remain resistant to cavities and there are no health consequences of fluorosis. Recently there has been an increase in dental fluorosis from increased exposure to fluoride through the additive effects of fluoridated water, fluoride supplements, foods and drinks made with fluoridated water, toothpaste and mouthwashes. Fluorosis is now seen in up to 60 percent of children.

RECOMMENDED SUPPLEMENTAL FLUORIDE CONCENTRATIONS FOR CHILDREN

Age of Child	Fluoride Concentration of Principal Drinking Water	
	◄ 0.3 ppm	► 0.3 ppm
0 to 6 mths	None	None
6 mths to 3 yrs	0.25 mg/day	None
3 to 6 yrs	0.5 mg/day	None
6 yrs	I mg/day	None

Source: Canadian Paediatric Society: *Paediatrics & Child Health 2002;* 7(8):569–572, Reference no. N02-01.

To determine the fluoride content of your water supply, contact your doctor, dentist or local water authority office.

OTHER FLUIDS Fruit juice is an excellent source of vitamin C, but should not be introduced until the second year to avoid it becoming a substitute for breast milk or infant formula. Furthermore, excessive juice intake may be a cause of failure to thrive or chronic diarrhea. If offering juice, do not dilute it with water. The recommended daily allowance of vitamin C for infants aged 6 to 12 months is 20mg/day and it is easily provided in breast milk, formula, fruits and vegetables. Babies less than one year may be offered water once they are well established on breast milk or formula and gaining weight well. They do not require extra water in addition to breast milk or formula except in hot weather.

COLIC Colic is defined as excessive crying in healthy infants that persists for at least 3 hours, on at least 3 days per week, for at least 3 weeks. Colic is thought to occur in approximately 13 percent of infants and usually begins at 3 to 4 weeks of age and persists until the infant is about 3 to 4 months of age. Although there are many theories, the cause of colic remains unknown, as does the cure.

When faced with excessive crying it is important to ask the following questions: Is baby hungry, cold, hot or in pain? Provided your baby is healthy, thriving and not found to have any abnormality on examination by your doctor, it is possible he may have colic. During crying spells both parents and baby endure significant stress. There are no medications or remedies that have been proven safe and effective to relieve crying. Parents are encouraged to try stroking, massaging, rocking and cuddling the infant. There is no evidence to support changing to soy formula to relieve colic; however, your doctor may suggest a week-long trial of a protein hydrosylate formula if baby is formula-fed.

As crying spells can be extremely upsetting to parents, it is important to request assistance from friends and relatives in caring for a baby with colic. If you ever feel "at the end of your rope," contact your doctor immediately.

WEANING Weaning is the introduction of foods other than breast milk. This may be whole cow's milk (if over 12 months) or formula (if exclusive breast feeding is no longer possible). Milk or formula will now be delivered by cup or bottle and will taste very different from breast milk. It is best to make the transition slowly to allow a smooth adjustment for both baby and parent. Weaning may begin by replacing the baby's least favorite feed per day with formula or whole cow's milk. For each subsequent week, replace an additional daily feed. This process may take 4 to 6 weeks or longer, depending on your baby.

BREAST MILK AND IMMUNIZATIONS

At the ages of 2, 4, 6, 12 and 18 months, your doctor will offer your baby immunizations. It has been recognized that breastfed babies may develop a stronger immunity to some diseases and are presumably better protected. This response is just one of the many benefits of breastfeeding and is thought to be because of the fatty acids present in breast milk. One of these fatty acids, linoleic acid, has recently been added to some infant formulas and improved immunity has also been seen in babies fed these formulas.

From Six Months

Your baby is showing an increased interest in the food you are eating, seems unsatisfied after feeds, and is waking up more in the night. You've also noticed that she's able to hold her head up and sit in an upright position.

The time has come: she's ready for solid food. Your *homemade* food.

PREPARING BABY FOOD

Making baby food is easy. To get started, all you need is the following:
- this book
- steamer basket (or multi-layer steamer)
- blender or food processor
- ice cube trays
- freezer bags and labels
- freezer
- small double-boiler
- plastic wrap
- and, of course, a hungry baby!

Steaming is the method of choice for cooking fruits and vegetables as it preserves their fresh taste, vitamin content and even color. You'll need a blender or food processor to purée the food to suit your baby's age and taste. Simply pour the puréed food into ice cube trays covered with plastic wrap, freeze, and later transfer the food cubes to labeled freezer bags. When your baby is hungry, preparing a meal is as easy as defrosting a cube.

Before you get started, here are a few things to keep in mind:

▶ *Hygiene:* Cleanliness is extremely important when preparing food for your family. Prior to making baby food, wash your hands thoroughly with soap and warm water, and ensure that the equipment and the cooking areas are clean. Equipment and utensils should be thoroughly hand washed using hot water and detergent, or cleaned in a dishwasher on a high heat setting. All fruits and vegetables, including those being peeled, should be thoroughly washed. This is because surface bacteria on the skin comes into contact with the knife or peeler.

▶ *Get fresh:* When making food for your baby, always use the freshest ingredients.

▶ *Do it right:* Always ensure that food is correctly cooked before freezing it or serving it to your baby.

▶ *Straining or puréeing:* Because of concerns about baby's choking, many experts advocate straining food for your infant's first few months. If your baby seems to be struggling with new textures, use a sieve: place 1/2 cup of cooked food in the sieve and press with the back of a spoon.

▶ *Freezing and storage:* After preparing any of the bulk recipes in *The Baby's Table,* pour the food into ice cube trays, cover with plastic wrap and freeze. Once cubes of food are frozen, they can be stored in airtight freezer bags. These should be carefully labeled and dated. Frozen baby food can be stored for up to 1 month in the freezer, and, once thawed, will keep for 48 hours in the refrigerator.

▶ *Thawing:* Baby food should always be thawed in the refrigerator, or in a double-boiler on the stovetop, never by leaving it out on the counter at room temperature. Proper thawing prevents the possibility of bacteria growing on the outer layer while the inner core is still frozen. Baby food does not need to be heated prior to serving. On summer days your baby may enjoy a chilled purée. If you choose to warm your baby's food, remember it should be no warmer than body temperature (37°C/98.6°F). This is because babies are used to the temperature of breast milk. Food can be warmed in either the double boiler that was used for defrosting or in a sauce pan over low heat. Before serving, remember to mix thoroughly and test in order to avoid hot spots. The most effective way to gauge the temperature of baby food is to test it yourself. Once food has been served, leftovers should be discarded because bacteria from the mouth will have contaminated the food. A microwave is not advised for warming as dangerous hot spots are much more likely to occur than with other methods of heating.

▶ *Cooking times and quantities:* For the recipes in this book, quantities are approximate and most are measured using a standard-size plastic ice cube tray. The number of cubes your baby will eat in a month varies depending on age, individual appetite and how often you choose to supplement the cubes. Supplemental foods include whole-grain infant cereals and finger foods (after 8 months). When your baby is 6 months old you might make only 2 recipes: 1 fruit and 1 vegetable. You will need 2 ice cube trays and it will take approximately 20 minutes. By the time your baby is 12 months old you may be making 4 to 6 recipes per month: 1 meat, 1 pasta, 1 fish and 2 vegetables. Depending on the complexity of the recipes and how many you make, it will take approximately 2 to 4 hours and you will probably need 6 to 8 ice cube trays. If you have a very hungry baby, be prepared to invest in additional ice cube trays. As your baby gets older, muffin tins work just as well and produce larger portions. Cooking times too will vary.

▶ *Allergy alert:* The recipes in the following chapters adhere to accepted guidelines for introducing foods to your baby at various stages so as to avoid or identify possible allergic reactions. For more information on allergies, see the sections Starting Solids and Food Allergies, next.

STARTING SOLIDS

The recommended age to start your baby on solid foods has changed dramatically over the years and between countries. Recommendations for the introduction of particular food groups have also varied considerably. Our recommendations in *The Baby's Table* are based on *Nutrition for Healthy Term Infants*, the statement of the Joint Working Group of the Canadian Paediatric Society, the Dietitians of Canada and Health Canada. These recommendations are based on two things: maximizing the time the infant spends exclusively breastfeeding, and ensuring the infant is physiologically mature enough to digest solid foods.

Ideally solids should be introduced to babies when they are 6 months old. Introducing food at this age is thought to minimize the

SIGNS YOUR BABY MAY BE READY TO START SOLID FOODS

• Baby is consistently waking more frequently in the night.
• Baby is interested in the foods you are eating.
• Baby seems unsatisfied after feeds.
• Baby frequently seems bored or disinterested in feeds.
• Baby is crying more often between feeds.
• Baby is falling off growth curves on plots of weight measurements.
• Baby is able to sit in an upright position and able to hold his head up.

risk of gastrointestinal infections. On the other hand, if parents wait until their infants are much older than 6 months to introduce solid foods, the baby runs the risk of developing iron-deficiency anemia as his fetal stores gradually become depleted.

Your baby, like every baby, is unique and will be ready to begin eating solids at a different time from your best friend's baby or the baby next door. Watch for the signs mentioned in the chart above. If your baby demonstrates these signs it may be acceptable to begin solids a little earlier. Consult your doctor if you suspect your baby is hungry and should begin eating solids before 6 months.

The first foods you should introduce are iron-fortified single-grain cereals, and there are no substitutes. These cereals are unlikely to cause allergies, are easily digested, and have been fortified to replenish iron stores. Iron-fortified infant cereals will form the basis of your baby's diet for the first 2 years of life, and will help to ensure adequate iron intake.

A good first choice is iron-fortified rice cereal followed at weekly intervals by barley, oatmeal and, finally, wheat. By introducing these foods one by one, you are more likely to identify any allergy your baby might have to a single grain. It is best to introduce wheat last as wheat is associated with increased incidence of allergies. After you have introduced all grains individually, you can start introducing mixed cereals.

Initial feedings are for practice and pleasure only. If your baby resists these first attempts, do not be disappointed. Try again another day. Breast milk or formula still constitute the majority of calories and nutrients, anyway, so only offer small amounts of solid food at a relaxed pace. Start with 1 tablespoon, mixed with breast milk or formula, and slowly increase the quantity as your baby desires. After the first week and depending on your baby's appetite, increase servings of rice cereal to twice daily. Always observe your baby's cues of satiety and hunger. Do not overfeed or persist if baby seems full or uninterested.

Once your baby has mastered rice cereal, you can begin to introduce fruits and vegetables. The decision to start vegetables or fruit first is controversial. Breast milk, formula and rice cereal are all quite sweet, and many think that a baby will naturally prefer the sweeter taste of fruit. So, in order to ensure they will accept vegetables, some believe they should be introduced before fruit. Others say it makes no difference and it's fine to start with either. Furthermore, a recent study suggests that childhood taste preferences are shaped by the sweetness of breastmilk or formula in the first few months of life. Most interestingly in breastfed babies, childhood preferences seem to resemble those of the mother in the early months of breastfeeding. Once again, there is a lot of "advice" about baby care but the best choice is usually the one that works well for you and your baby.

Most fruits and vegetables can be cooked in bulk, puréed to a fine consistency and then frozen. When introducing a new food, serve it either on its own or with familiar foods—again, to monitor for adverse reactions such as diarrhea, rash or constipation.

At 6 to 8 months of age infants are learning how to bite, chew and swallow. You can encourage your baby by gradually introducing a variety of new foods with different textures. Poultry, red meat and pasta may now be offered.

By 8 months of age your baby has been exposed to an array of foods. At this stage, the recipes you can prepare become more complex and involve combinations of several food groups. Fish and dairy products may now be added (with the exception of whole cow's milk for drinking, which should be postponed until at least 12 months of age). At 1 year of age, babies can start eating eggs. General recommendations apply to infants without a family history of food allergy, and certain foods must always be avoided in infancy (see the chart entitled Proceed with Caution on page 57).

ADVERSE REACTIONS AND ALLERGIES

In babies and toddlers most symptoms caused by foods are not allergic reactions, but are called "adverse reactions to foods" or "food intolerances." These reactions most commonly occur in the first year of life and disappear by 3 years of age. Approximately one-third of all children will have an adverse reaction to food characterized by any of the following: vomiting, diarrhea, skin rashes, itching, runny nose, congestion or wheezing. Adverse reactions may also occur from exposure to additives such as artificial flavors and colors.

Food allergies or "food hypersensitivity" occur much less commonly, affecting only 8 percent of children less than 1 year of age. Almost half of the children who develop a food allergy by age 3 will outgrow it. True food allergy is present in only 1 to 2 percent of adults. Food allergy occurs when the immune system mistakenly tries to defend the body against food proteins (allergens) by producing antibodies. Usually repeated exposure to the food is required to produce enough antibodies to produce an allergic reaction—a process called sensitization. Eventually, exposure to the food results in enough antibodies to produce allergic symptoms. These symptoms range from runny nose, itchy eyes and skin rash to anaphylaxis: a rare condition of mouth or throat swelling,

25

difficulty in breathing and/or collapse and shock. Symptoms may occur within minutes or up to 72 hours after ingestion of the allergen. Anaphylaxis is a life-threatening emergency: seek medical attention immediately.

Anaphylaxis most notably occurs to peanuts and usually persists into adulthood. All children should be at least 18 months old before being offered peanuts, including peanut butter and other peanut products. Any child diagnosed with a severe food allergy should always have caregivers who are informed and prepared to manage an anaphylactic reaction and should be fitted with a MedicAlert bracelet listing food allergies. Doctors usually recommend that children keep with them a dose of epinephrine in an easy-to-use "pen" injector. Should anaphylaxis occur, the medication should be administered immediately prior to the onset of respiratory symptoms. Fatalities have occurred when children are inadvertently given the food and medication was not administered immediately.

Peanut, soy, tree nuts (for example, hazelnut, walnut, almond and cashew), wheat, cow's milk, strawberries, fish and eggs cause 95 percent of all food allergies. Fortunately it is very rare for children to have serious allergies to more than two or three foods. Diagnosis of allergy requires a careful analysis of the diet and symptoms and, if necessary, specific tests to confirm allergy rather than the much more common "food intolerance." If tests are positive for food allergy, your doctor will recommend removing the offending food from the diet, and having the child take a subsequent medically supervised challenge test at a later date—at which point it is very possible the child will have outgrown the allergy.

CAN FOOD ALLERGIES BE AVOIDED? Development of food allergy depends on genetic predisposition. If there is a family history of food allergies it is more likely that your child may develop one. Your doctor may recommend modifications to the regular introduction of solids if there is a chance of food allergy based on family history. As these foods are important sources of nutrition and difficult to avoid, always discuss the necessity to postpone them with your doctor. True diagnosis of allergy is difficult, and what may be remembered as an "allergy" by family members may have been the much more common "food intolerance."

Cow's milk allergy is the most common food allergy among young children. The introduction of cow's milk should be postponed until 12 months of age in all babies. Cow's milk dairy products such as yogurt and cheese may be introduced earlier, at 8 months. If your child is thought to be at risk of cow's milk allergy, your doctor may advise no cow's milk dairy products (for example, yogurt and cheese) until at least 12 months of age. Exclusive breastfeeding for at least 4 to 6 months has been shown to minimize the risk of developing allergies in those infants with a family history. If formula-feeding, whey-protein hydrosylate formula is a better alternative to cow's milk protein–based formula for infants at risk for milk allergy. Soy formula should not be used as it is also possible to develop an allergy to soy. Fortunately, the vast majority of children outgrow cow's milk allergy by age 3 or 4.

Whole eggs should be postponed until 1 year of age but well-cooked egg yolk may be introduced after 9 months. If there is a family history of food allergies, consult with your doctor regarding postponing eggs beyond that point. Avoiding eggs means avoiding "egg substitutes" and any foods that list albumin, globulin, ovomucin or vitellin. Egg products were once used in the production of the MMR (measles, mumps and rubella) vaccine, although newer versions of the vaccine are egg-product free. Flu shots also contain egg products. Although allergic reactions to vaccines are very rare, always advise your doctor prior to vaccination if there is an egg allergy or family history of food allergies.

Wheat is the most common grain allergy. In all babies, it is best to delay introducing wheat until other grain cereals have been introduced. Wheat is a "hidden" ingredient in many foods such as processed cheese and battered fish sticks, and careful analysis of ingredients is required to avoid it.

If advised to avoid or postpone feeding your baby certain foods you should be aware of all foods that may contain it. Full lists of all hidden sources, food labeling and safe alternatives can be obtained from The American Academy of Allergy, Asthma and Immunology (see Appendix I).

To diagnose true food allergy or for management of complex or multiple allergies, consult with a pediatric allergist and pediatric dietitian.

FRUIT

From single fruit mash to mixed fruit smoothies, fruit will likely be a hit with baby. Fruit is an important source of many vitamins and minerals, and the high level of vitamin C in many fruits promotes healthy growth of skin and bones, and facilitates iron absorption. Babies also find fruit easy to digest. Best of all, the natural sugars appeal to their developing tastebuds.

It is important to choose well-ripened fruit, which is sweet. All fruits, with the exception of banana and avocado, are easier to eat if steamed. It is advisable to postpone citrus fruits until after 1 year due to their high acidity. After cooking, purée the fruit in a food processor until smooth. Very young babies prefer their food to be almost liquid. You can accomplish this by adding some leftover cooking water, unsweetened apple juice, breast milk or formula. When adding liquid, mix in a tablespoon at a time to achieve desired consistency. All cooked fruit can be made in bulk and then frozen.

Breastfed babies tend to be slightly leaner than formula-fed infants; however, they catch up once solids are established. The difference in growth rates is likely because of the difference in fat and protein contents of breast milk and formula. Breast milk adapts to baby's age and to climate, to provide adequate nutrition depending on growth and caloric needs. This difference is entirely normal and expected provided your baby is growing and thriving. Plot your baby's height and weight on a standardized growth curve to follow his development through the first year (see Appendix II, page 161).

BANANAS

Typically, banana is the first raw fruit you will feed your baby. Once the infant is ready to move on, banana blends well with other fruits (because of its creamy texture) to make delicious fruit combinations. Try mixing mashed banana with a cube of your baby's favorite fruit purée.

1/4 banana, skin removed
1 tbsp breast milk or formula
(approx)

• In bowl, mash banana with fork to remove lumps. Add breast milk or formula (if needed) to make banana more appealing for younger babies. Serve immediately to prevent banana from turning brown. Once mashed, banana should not be frozen.

Yield: 1 serving

FROM SIX MONTHS

APPLES

When choosing apples, remember the sweeter the better; try Golden Delicious or Fuji.

6 medium apples, washed, peeled, cored and quartered

• In steamer, steam apples over boiling water for 10 minutes. Set leftover cooking water aside.
• In a blender or food processor, purée until smooth. For very young babies you may choose to add leftover cooking water to thin out the purée. When thinning, add 1 tbsp of liquid at a time.
• Pour into ice cube trays and freeze.

Yield: 10 to 12 cubes

PEARS

6 medium pears, washed, peeled, cored and quartered

• In steamer, steam pears over boiling water for 8 minutes.
• In blender or food processor, purée until smooth, adding leftover cooking water if needed.
• Pour into ice cube trays and freeze.

Yield: 10 to 12 cubes

MELON

1 medium-size cantaloupe or honeydew melon, washed

• Cut melon in half, remove seeds and scoop out fruit.
• In steamer, steam over boiling water for 6 minutes.
• In blender or food processor, purée until smooth.
• Pour into ice cube trays and freeze.

Yield: 6 to 8 cubes

QUANTITIES

The majority of the recipes in this book do not require exact measurements. This flexibility eliminates the concern of having to measure exactly. The quantities of liquid required are approximate. This enables you to meet your baby's changing preferences. Young babies like their food runny and puréed to a fine consistency. As your baby matures, she will be able to handle lumpier textures that require less liquid.

PEACHES

The following recipe is also tasty made with nectarines, plums or apricots.

4 peaches, washed

• In a pot of boiling water, plunge peaches for 2 minutes. Remove from water and allow to cool.
• Slit skin with a knife and peel. Cut peach into quarters and remove pit. In steamer, steam fruit over boiling water for 4 minutes.
• In blender or food processor, purée until smooth.
• Pour into ice cube trays and freeze.

Yield: 8 to 10 cubes

PAPAYA

Papaya mixes well with banana. To prepare, defrost 1 cube of papaya and mix with 1/4 mashed banana. Adding 1 tbsp of milk (breast or formula) will help to thin out the purée, making it more palatable for baby. Serve at room temperature.

I medium-size papaya, washed

• Cut papaya in half, remove seeds and scoop out fruit.
• In steamer, steam fruit over boiling water for 6 minutes.
• In blender or food processor, purée until smooth.
• Pour into ice cube trays and freeze.

Yield: 6 cubes

SHOULD YOU USE THE MICROWAVE FOR BABY FOOD PREPARATION?

There has been recent controversy over the use of microwaves for food preparation. Concerns have been raised over the potential of microwaves to alter the composition of breast milk, to destroy valuable nutrients in food and to possibly leach toxins from cooking containers. We advise that the microwave never be used to heat baby milk (breast milk or formula) or to warm baby food, in order to avoid dangerous hotspots and the possible disruption of breast milk antibodies. A recent study found that microwaving broccoli can leach its cancer-fighting properties, while microwaving a potato actually preserves nutrients when compared to cooking it in a conventional oven. We therefore advise using a conventional stove for all meat, fish, pasta and vegetable preparation, with the exception of baked potatoes in the toddler section—these may be microwaved if desired.

FRUIT TRIO

This recipe can be made with any combination of either the fruit purées or mashed banana. Experiment to find out which combinations your baby most enjoys!

I cube pear purée
I cube apple purée
I cube cantaloupe purée

• Defrost fruit cubes, mix in bowl and serve at room temperature.

Yield: 1 serving

CINNAMON APPLES

FRUIT CEREAL

On a hot summer's day, mash frozen apple cubes with equal parts baby cereal and serve when thawed but still cool.

Once your baby is comfortable eating a variety of fruit purées, you may want to try a little spice. Cinnamon, a delicious addition to both apple and pear, is a good one to start with. Remember to add the cinnamon before you steam the fruit. However, if you have a family history of allergies, delay the introduction of cinnamon until after baby is 9 months old.

I cube fruit purée (apple or pear
   is ideal to start with)
I tbsp single-grain baby cereal
   (start with rice)
2 tbsp breast milk or formula
   (approx)

6 medium apples, washed,
   peeled, cored and quartered
I/4 tsp cinnamon

• Defrost fruit purée.
• Combine rice with breast milk or formula to make baby rice.
• In saucepan mix rice and fruit together and warm. If combination seems too thick, add extra milk as needed.

• Sprinkle cinnamon on apples. In steamer, steam over boiling water for 10 minutes.
• In a blender or food processor, purée to desired consistency.
•Pour into ice cube trays and freeze.

Yield: 1 serving

Yield: 10 to 12 cubes

MASHED AVOCADO

Avocados are one of the few fruits that contain the essential monounsaturated fats. They are rich in potassium and also contain vitamins B, C and E. Introduce avocados early so your baby will learn to love them.

I avocado, washed
I tbsp breast milk or formula
   (approx)

• Cut avocado in half. Remove pit and scoop out flesh.
• In bowl, mash avocado with a fork, removing lumps. If mixture seems too thick, add milk as needed. Serve immediately to prevent avocado from turning brown. Leftover avocado can be frozen in ice cube trays.
• *To serve:* Defrost and serve at room temperature.

Yield: 3 to 4 cubes

FLORIDA BREAKFAST

I cube pear purée
1/4 mashed banana
I tbsp breast milk or formula
   (approx)

• Defrost pear purée and mix with mashed banana and milk. Serve immediately to prevent banana from turning brown.

Yield: 1 serving

34

VEGETABLES

Vegetables are rich in the vitamins, minerals and carbohydrates your growing baby needs. Although most commonly associated with vitamins, vegetables should also be valued for their high mineral content, most notably calcium, iron and zinc.

The root vegetables are naturally sweet and so they are a good place to start. Mixing these root vegetables with the stronger tasting green vegetables will make them more palatable. Initially your baby will require runny purées. Mix some leftover cooking water, unsweetened apple juice or homemade vegetable stock (recipe, page 41) into the purée. Add 1 tablespoon at a time to achieve the desired consistency. As with fruit, all of the following purées can be made in bulk and frozen.

WHOLE FOOD VERSUS SUPPLEMENTS

An entire day's supply of vitamin C can be obtained from either an apple or a vitamin supplement. However, the natural source is superior as it provides not only the needed vitamin C but also calcium, fiber and simple carbohydrates for energy. Many whole foods also contain phytochemicals, which have been linked to potential protective effects against cancer, heart disease, osteoporosis and diabetes. Phytochemicals, such as beta-carotene and lypocene, are substances derived from plants. Whole foods lay a healthy foundation for your baby's future.

BENEFITS OF BETA-CAROTENE

Beta-carotene is a phytochemical that acts as an antioxidant and thereby reduces the risk of some cancers in adults. It is found in yellow, orange and red fruits and vegetables. Studies have indicated it may help to reduce heart disease and improve arthritis in adults—and research is continuing. Although supplements are available, their long-term safety has not been adequately studied. For now, the best sources of beta carotene are carrots, pumpkin, squash, sweet potatoes, cantaloupe, mango and papaya. It is possible for babies to eat an excess of beta-carotene and develop a harmless condition called hypercarotenemia, characterized by an orange pigmentation of the skin and hair. Remember, it is better to provide your baby with a wide variety of fruits and vegetables.

SWEET POTATO

This naturally sweet vegetable is always a hit with babies. Sweet potato and apple make a delicious combination. Defrost 1 cube apple purée and 1 cube sweet potato purée. Mix and serve at room temperature.

2 sweet potatoes, washed,
    peeled, blemishes removed,
    cut in cubes

• In saucepan, bring potatoes to a boil, turn down the heat and simmer until tender, 20 to 30 minutes. Drain potatoes and set leftover cooking water aside.
• Place potatoes in blender or food processor and purée, adding leftover cooking water as needed to achieve desired consistency.
• Pour into ice cube trays and freeze.

Yield: 12 cubes

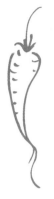

CARROT

Baby carrots are best as they are sweeter and are more likely to appeal.

8 baby carrots, washed, peeled, and sliced

• In steamer, steam carrots over boiling water for 15 minutes. Set leftover cooking water aside.
• In blender or food processor, purée until smooth, adding leftover cooking water as needed.
• Pour into ice cube trays and freeze.

Yield: 8 to 10 cubes

SWEETEN UP THE DEAL!

If your baby rejects a new vegetable, don't get discouraged. Mixing the vegetable with a favorite fruit may make it more appealing. Carrots, for example, mix well with either pear or apple. As your baby becomes more comfortable with the new vegetable, decrease the proportion of fruit and increase the vegetable. Be flexible and experiment to find out which combinations your baby most enjoys.

CARROT APPLE DELIGHT

2 cubes apple purée
I cube carrot purée

• Defrost the purées. In bowl, mix thoroughly and serve at room temperature.

Yield: 1 serving

LUSCIOUS YAMS

4 yams, washed, peeled and
   blemishes removed
1/2 cup of leftover cooking water
   (approx)

• Cut the yams into cubes.
• In steamer, cook yams over boiling water until tender, about 20 minutes. Set leftover cooking water aside.
• In blender or food processor, purée yams, adding leftover cooking water as needed to achieve desired consistency.
• Pour into ice cube trays and freeze.

Yield: 19 to 20 cubes

BUTTERNUT SQUASH

Butternut squash is naturally sweet and another vegetable that will probably make your baby's top ten favorite foods list.

I butternut squash, washed

• Peel skin using a sharp paring knife. Cut squash in half, remove seeds and section.
• In steamer, cook over boiling water until tender, 10 to 12 minutes. Set leftover cooking water aside.
• In blender or food processor, purée squash until smooth, adding leftover cooking water if needed.
• Pour into ice cube trays and freeze.

Yield: 10 cubes

FROM SIX MONTHS

POTATO

Because of their texture, potatoes mix very well with other vegetables. Try them combined with a cube of either broccoli or green bean purée.

I potato, washed, peeled and
    blemishes removed
1/2 cup breast milk or formula

• In saucepan of boiling water, cook potatoes until tender, about 20 minutes. (Boiling is quicker and often more convenient than baking; however, baking preserves more of the potato's nutrients. To bake, prick skin with a fork. Place potato in oven at 400°F for 1 hour.) To microwave, prick skin with a fork. Place potato in microwave on high for 4 to 6 minutes.
• In bowl, mash cooked potato with fork, or in blender or food processor, purée. Add milk to achieve desired consistency.
• Pour into ice cube trays and freeze.

Yield: 6 cubes

GREEN BEANS

2 handfuls green beans, washed,
    ends and stringy bits removed

• In steamer, cook beans over boiling water for 10 to 12 minutes. Set leftover cooking water aside.
• In blender or food processor, purée until smooth, adding leftover cooking water if needed.
• Pour into ice cube trays and freeze.

Yield: 6 cubes

BROCCOLI FIGHTS CANCER

Broccoli, rich in both calcium and iron, also contains phytochemicals known as isothiocyanates. These isothiocyanates have been shown to retard cancer cell growth in research studies. This may explain why people who eat broccoli regularly tend to have a lower risk of colon cancer. Whether these benefits extend to babies and children is not yet known. As colon cancer is the third most common cancer in North America, broccoli is an excellent investment in your baby's future. Introduce it early and serve it frequently.

BROCCOLI

This purée can be made with either broccoli or cauliflower. As broccoli has a rather strong taste, try combining it with potato when introducing it for the first time. To make, defrost 1 cube potato purée and 1 cube broccoli purée. In bowl, mix and serve at room temperature.

I bunch broccoli, washed and cut
  in florets

• In steamer, cook over boiling water until tender, 10 to 15 minutes. Set leftover cooking water aside.
• In blender or food processor, purée until smooth, adding leftover cooking water if needed.
• Pour into ice cube trays and freeze.

Yield: 10 to 12 cubes

40

VEGETABLE STOCK

Vegetable stock can be used instead of the leftover cooking water to thin out purées. The following recipes call for vegetable stock; however, its use is optional as leftover cooking water can be substituted with adequate results. Stock enhances both the taste and nutritional value of the dish.

I leek, washed, sections separated
   and sliced
I parsnip, washed, peeled and sliced
4 stalks celery including leaves,
   washed, trimmed and sliced
4 carrots, washed, peeled and sliced
I potato, washed, peeled and cut
   in cubes
I onion, cut in chunks
2 sprigs fresh parsley
I bay leaf
I sprig fresh rosemary
10 cups water
4 peppercorns

• In large pot of water, place vegetables, herbs and peppercorns; bring to a rapid boil. Turn down heat and simmer, partially covered, until vegetables have released their flavor, about 3 to 4 hours.
• Strain and discard vegetables.
• Pour stock into ice cube trays and freeze.

Yield: 32 cubes

VEGETABLE RICE

When making this recipe for the first time, start with either carrot or sweet potato.

I cube vegetable purée
I tbsp single-grain baby cereal
   (start with rice)
2 tbsp breast milk or formula
   (approx)

• Defrost vegetable purée.
• Combine rice with 2 tbsp breast milk or formula to make baby rice.
• In saucepan, mix rice and vegetables together and warm over low heat. If combination seems too thick, add extra milk as needed.

Yield: 1 serving

BABY BUNNY'S PURÉE

This tasty concoction will have your little bunny wanting more.

3 carrots, washed, peeled and
   sliced
3 parsnips, washed, peeled and
   sliced
1/4 cup Vegetable Stock (2 to 3
   cubes) (recipe, page 41)
or
leftover cooking water (optional)

• In steamer, cook vegetables over boiling water for 15 minutes.
• In blender or food processor, purée until smooth, adding stock (if needed) to achieve desired consistency.
• Pour into ice cube trays and freeze.

Yield: 8 to 10 cubes

VEGETABLE TRIO

1 potato, washed, peeled and cut
   in cubes
1 carrot, washed, peeled and
   sliced
1/4 bunch broccoli, washed and
   cut in florets
1/4 cup Vegetable Stock (2 to 3
   cubes) (recipe, page 41)
or
leftover cooking water (optional)

• In saucepan of boiling water, cook potato until tender, about 20 minutes.
• In steamer, steam remaining vegetables until tender, about 15 minutes.
• In blender or food processor, purée vegetables, adding stock (if needed) to achieve desired consistency.
• Pour into ice cube trays and freeze.

Yield 12 to 14 cubes

WHAT ABOUT NITRATES?

At one time it was recommended that home-prepared carrots, spinach, turnip and beets not be fed to very young infants. The level of nitrates, compared to that in commercially processed vegetables (which removes some nitrates), could be detrimental to the infant kidney. However, now that it is customary to introduce solids at the later age of 6 months, current recommendations do not advise restricting these nutritious vegetables. Nitrates are not a concern for healthy term infants over 4 months of age.

BROCCOLI, WATERCRESS AND POTATO

1/3 bunch broccoli, washed and
    cut in florets
I potato, washed and baked
2 handfuls fresh watercress, thor-
    oughly washed, stalks removed
1/4 cup Vegetable Stock (2 to 3
    cubes) (recipe, page 41)
or
leftover cooking water (optional)

• Peel potato and cut in cubes.
• In steamer, cook broccoli over boiling water until tender, about 15 minutes; add watercress for last 3 minutes of cooking time.
• In blender or food processor, purée potato and broccoli mixture until smooth, adding stock (if needed) to achieve desired consistency.
• Pour into ice cube trays and freeze.

Yield: 10 to 12 cubes

HOW MUCH CALCIUM?

Ninety-nine percent of the body's skeleton is made up of calcium. During rapid growth in the first 2 years of life it is essential to provide your baby with sufficient calcium to optimize growth potential and to build strong bones. Despite high breast milk or infant formula intake over this period, some babies fail to meet recommended daily intakes of calcium. Furthermore, recommended intakes of calcium increase significantly throughout the first 2 years to reflect the increasing demands of growth. To increase your baby's calcium levels, offer vegetables naturally high in calcium such as bok choy, broccoli and watercress.

OPTIMAL CALCIUM REQUIREMENTS

AGE	RECOMMENDED CALCIUM INTAKE
0-6 mths	210 mg/day
6-12 mths	270 mg/day
1-3 yrs	500 mg/day
4-8 yrs	800 mg/day
9-18 yrs	1500 mg/day
Pregnancy or breastfeeding	
18 and younger	1300 mg/day
19-50 yrs	1000 mg/day

CALCIUM CONTENT OF SELECTED FOODS

FOOD	SERVING	CALCIUM (mg)
Milk	250 ml (1 cup)	315
Firm cheese	50 g (1.6 oz)	350
Yogurt	125 ml (1/2 cup)	196
Baked beans	250 ml (1 cup)	163
Bok choy, cooked	125 ml (1/2 cup)	84
Broccoli, cooked	125 ml (1/2 cup)	38
Chick-peas, cooked	250 ml (1 cup)	84
Orange	1 medium	52
Rhubarb, cooked	125 ml (1/2 cup)	184
Salmon, canned	1/2 213-g can (7 oz)	225
Sardines, canned	1/2 213-g can (7 oz)	210

Source: Standing Committee on the Scientific Evaluation of Dietary Reference Intakes, Food and Nutrition Board, Institute of Medicine, 1997.

CALCIUM CRUNCH

I potato, washed and baked

1/3 bunch broccoli, washed and
cut in florets

4 bunches baby bok choy, outer
layers removed, trimmed and
washed between leaves

• Peel potato and cut in chunks.
• In steamer, cook broccoli over boiling water until tender, about 15 minutes. Remove broccoli. Place bok choy in steamer; steam until tender, 4 to 5 minutes. Set aside leftover cooking water.
• Place vegetables in food processor and purée until smooth. If purée seems too thick, add leftover cooking water as needed, 1 tbsp at a time.
• Pour into ice cube trays and freeze.

Yield: 14 to 16 cubes

VEGGIE DELIGHT

I potato, washed, peeled and cut
in cubes

I zucchini, washed, trimmed and
sliced

1/4 bunch broccoli, washed and
cut in florets

1/3 cup Vegetable Stock (3 to 4
cubes) (recipe, page 4I)

or

leftover cooking water (optional)

• In saucepan of boiling water, cook potato until tender, about 20 minutes.
• In steamer, cook zucchini and broccoli over boiling water until tender, about 15 minutes.
• In blender or food processor, purée vegetables until smooth, adding vegetable stock (if needed) to achieve desired consistency.
• Pour into ice cube trays and freeze.

Yield: 10 to 12 cubes

RETHINKING FAT FOR BABIES

In today's health-conscious society adults place great emphasis on reducing fat and cholesterol intake in an effort to prevent heart disease and control weight. Such restrictions, however, can be dangerous when applied to infants under 2 years of age. During this time of rapid growth, fats are used as a dense source of calories for energy and constitute a major part of the developing brain. Unlike with adults, there is no evidence that restricting fats in babies prevents disease later in life. For this reason, the Canadian Paediatric Society recommends that fats constitute approximately 50 percent of the infant's diet until the age of 2. The majority of this fat is obtained from breast milk or infant formula, followed by milk. As your child grows, the need for fats diminishes and lower-fat choices may be appropriate. Until 2 years, however, baby needs whole-fat dairy products. Do not place your baby on a low-fat diet unless advised by your doctor.

WHAT ARE TRANS FATS?

A high-fat diet is essential for optimal growth and development in the first 2 years of life. Fat intake ensures proper brain and nerve development and supplies energy for growth. This fat is available in whole foods, most notably breast milk, dairy, meats and oils.

There are four kinds of fats: monounsaturated fat, polyunsaturated fat, saturated fat and trans fat. Monounsaturated fats and polyunsaturated fats are considered good fats. Saturated fats are found in meat, dairy and some vegetables and include butter, shortening, animal fat, palm oil and coconut oil. Trans fats are dangerous fats and contribute to diabetes, heart disease, immune disfunction and obesity in adults. There is no safe amount of these fats and they have been labeled the biggest food-processing disaster in history. Trans fats are placed in processed foods to prolong shelf life; they have no nutritional value. Packaging and labelling laws do not require that trans fats be identified in the ingredients, so stay away from any foods which list "partially hydrogenated" or trans-fat to be safe. To avoid the risks of these fats be sure to live by the whole food philosophy.

CHICKEN

Although both red meat and chicken can be introduced from 6 months, chicken is the natural first choice. It is an excellent source of protein for muscle development and energy. It also contains omega-6 fatty acids, which are essential for brain growth and development. Mixing chicken with one of your baby's favourite fruits or vegetables is the best way to ensure its acceptance. If rejected, put the chicken away and try again another day. Research indicates it may take as many as 10–15 exposures before a new food is accepted. The development of healthy life-long eating habits takes persistence and dedication, but these habits may have lasting implications on your baby's future health.

Poaching is the ideal way to cook chicken for your baby. This method tenderizes the meat while it cooks and also eliminates the possibility of charring that can occur with grilling or broiling. Charred food contains known carcinogens and should be avoided. Adding a little leftover poaching water is an ideal way to thin out your chicken purées.

POACHED CHICKEN BREAST

Use this recipe as the basis for the puréed chicken recipes that follow.

1/2 chicken breast
I sprig fresh tarragon (optional)

• In a shallow frying pan, place chicken breast flat and add water to cover and tarragon (if using). Bring water to a boil, then cover pan with foil and reduce heat to a simmer for 5 minutes. Flip breast and continue to simmer for another 5 to 7 minutes, depending on the size of the breast. Allow chicken to cool in water. The meat should be firm to touch and white throughout. There should be no trace of pink and juices should run clear.

CHICKEN AND YAMS

I large yam, washed, peeled and
   cubed
1/2 Poached Chicken Breast
   (recipe p. 48)
1/4 cup leftover poaching water

• In steamer, steam yam over boiling water until tender, about 20 minutes.
• Chop chicken. In blender or food processor, purée chicken, yam and poaching water. If purée seems too thick, add extra poaching water to achieve desired consistency.
• Pour into ice cube trays and freeze.

Yield 14 cubes

CHICKEN APPLE DELIGHT

2 sweet apples, washed, peeled
and quartered
1/2 Poached Chicken Breast
(recipe, page 48)
2 tbsp unsweetened apple juice
(approx)

• In steamer, steam apples over boiling water for 10 minutes. In blender or food processor, purée chicken, apples and unsweetened apple juice to achieve desired consistency. If the purée seems too thick, add a little more apple juice as needed.
• Pour into ice cube trays and freeze.

Yield: 10 cubes

MAKE USE OF BABY'S LOVE OF THE SWEET

Babies tend to have an innate preference for sweet-tasting foods, and this preference can be used to introduce new flavors and textures. For example, introduce a new meat combined with baby's favorite fruit. Most of the chicken purées described may be combined with puréed apple to make a naturally sweeter version. If your baby rejects a new meat, don't get discouraged. Combine the purée with apple and serve at a later date.

SAMPLE MEAL PLANNER: FROM SIX MONTHS OF AGE

WEEK I

Breakfast	Breast or Bottle, Single-Grain Baby Cereal (Rice)
Mid-A.M. Snack	Breast or Bottle
Lunch	Breast or Bottle
Mid-P.M. Snack	Breast or Bottle
Dinner	Single-Grain Baby Cereal if desired
Before Bed	Breast or Bottle

WEEK 3

Breakfast	Breast or Bottle, Single-Grain Baby Cereal (Barley)
Mid-A.M. Snack	Breast or Bottle
Lunch	Breast or Bottle
Mid-P.M. Snack	Breast or Bottle
Dinner	Mashed Avocado or Butternut Squash
Before Bed	Breast or Bottle

WEEK 2

Breakfast	Breast or Bottle, Fruit Cereal
Mid-A.M. Snack	Breast or Bottle
Lunch	Breast or Bottle
Mid-P.M. Snack	Breast or Bottle
Dinner	Banana, Puréed Fruit or Sweet Potato
Before Bed	Breast or Bottle

WEEK 4

Breakfast	Breast or Bottle, Fruit Cereal
Mid-A.M. Snack	Breast or Bottle
Lunch	Breast or Bottle
Mid-P.M. Snack	Breast or Bottle
Dinner	Chicken and Yams
Before Bed	Breast or Bottle

Baby may also wake for additional feeds during the night.

You may mix any of the purées with baby cereal for palatability and increased iron.

FROM SIX MONTHS

SAMPLE MEAL PLANNER: SIX TO SEVEN MONTHS OF AGE

WEEK 5

Breakfast	Breast or Bottle, Fruit Cereal
Mid-A.M. Snack	Breast or Bottle
Lunch	Breast or Bottle, Mashed Banana (if desired)
Mid-P.M. Snack	Breast or Bottle
Dinner	Carrot or Potato
Before Bed	Breast or Bottle

WEEK 6

Breakfast	Breast or Bottle, Single-Grain Baby Cereal (Oats or Barley)
Mid-A.M. Snack	Breast or Bottle
Lunch	Breast or Bottle, Fruit Cereal (if desired)
Mid-P.M. Snack	Breast or Bottle
Dinner	Baby Bunny Purée or Vegetable Rice
Before Bed	Breast or Bottle

WEEK 7

Breakfast	Breast or Bottle, Single-Grain Baby Cereal (Oats or Barley)
Mid-A.M. Snack	Breast or Bottle
Lunch	Breast or Bottle, Carrot Apple Delight (if desired)
Mid-P.M. Snack	Breast or Bottle
Dinner	Vegetable Trio or Butternut Squash
Before Bed	Breast or Bottle

WEEK 8

Breakfast	Breast or Bottle, Fruit Cereal
Mid-A.M. Snack	Breast or Bottle
Lunch	Florida Breakfast
Mid-P.M. Snack	Breast or Bottle
Dinner	Chicken Apple Delight
Before Bed	Breast or Bottle

Baby may also wake for additional feeds during the night.

You may mix any of the purées with baby cereal for palatability and increased iron.

From Seven Months

It is never too early to set the foundation for a positive relationship with food and healthy lifelong eating habits. The best way to do this is to make sure that mealtimes are enjoyable for everyone. Although your baby will still need to be spoon-fed, it is not too early to encourage participation. While you are feeding her, place a tiny amount of purée in a bowl and allow her to explore. Although this may mean your precious purée will end up on the floor, be smushed in tiny hands or smeared on the serving tray, your baby will be grinning from ear to ear. Most messes can be minimized. Invest in a large bib and a suitable baby bowl. Don't get discouraged—this is a valuable learning experience. Once your baby begins to suck her fingers, she will learn that bringing her hand to her mouth results in tasty treats. When she is able to grasp a spoon, encourage her to hold her own during feedings. At first the spoon will just be waved in the air or banged on the tray, but slowly she will learn to dip and suck, just as she did with her fingers. Not only will your baby enjoy these initial steps toward independence, she will be distracted and it will be easier for you to spoon-feed the main course.

If your baby rejects a new purée or even a familiar favorite, don't push the issue. However nutritious the meal may be, it is not worth a power struggle, especially one you are unlikely to win. With a smile on your face, take the purée away and try again another day. The most important thing is that the meal end on a happy note for everyone.

FRUIT

By the age of 7 months your baby is able to eat uncooked fruit. It is important to serve well-ripened fruit as it is sweeter and easier on the digestive system. All fruits must be thoroughly washed and peeled. The softer fruits, such as pears, papaya, peaches and melons, are the obvious first choices as they are easily mashed with a fork. After mashing they can be mixed with unsweetened fruit juice, breast milk or formula to achieve a desired consistency. Mixing any combination of fresh fruit with a little unsweetened apple juice can make a delicious fruit salad. Oranges and other citrus fruits are acidic, however, and should not be introduced until after 12 months.

Though fresh fruit is best, you can introduce canned fruit if packed in its own juices with no added sugar. Dried fruit is rich in iron and has a high fiber content that functions as a natural laxative. Prior to age 8 months, baby's dried fruit should be stewed for 25 minutes and then puréed. After age 8 months, his dried fruit can be offered as a snack. As dried fruit has a concentrated sugar content it is important to clean baby's teeth afterward. This can be done with either a damp washcloth or a baby toothbrush, depending on the infant's age.

BABY'S FIRST FRUIT SALAD

1/4 small papaya, washed, both skin
    and seeds removed

1/4 avocado, washed and skin
    removed

I tbsp breast milk or formula
    (approx)

• In small bowl, mash avocado and papaya together with a fork. If mixture seems too thick, add milk to achieve desired consistency.

Yield: 1 serving

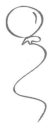

GROWTH AND DEVELOPMENT

Growth patterns of babies vary depending on multiple factors, such as genetic endowment, gestational age at birth, activity level and race. They also differ in the timing of individual growth spurts. Serial measurements of height, weight and head circumference are much more indicative of growth pattern than is a single measurement. Plot your baby's height, weight and head circumference on a standardized graph (see Appendix II). Provided your baby is following a smooth growth curve and is thriving, growth is likely occurring at your baby's own pace. Here are some approximate measurements:

RULES OF THUMB FOR GROWTH

WEIGHT, HEIGHT AND HEAD CIRCUMFERENCE

WEIGHT

Weight loss in first few days of life:	5 to 10% of birth weight
Return to birth weight:	7 to 10 days of life
Double birth weight:	4 to 5 months
Average birth weight:	3.5 kg (7.7 lbs)
Average weight at 1 year:	10 kg (22 lbs)
Average weight at 5 years:	20 kg (44 lbs)

HEIGHT

Average length at birth:	50 cm (19.7 inches)
Average height at 3 years:	90 cm (35.4 inches)
Average height at 4 years:	100 cm (39.3 inches), double birth length

HEAD CIRCUMFERENCE

Average head circumference at birth: 35 cm (13.8 inches)
Average head circumference increase: 2 cm (0.8 inch) per month for the first 3 months, then 1 cm (0.4 inch) per month from 4 to 12 months

DRIED FRUIT PURÉE

The flavor of this purée is quite rich. After age 8 months babies can eat it mixed with cottage cheese or yogurt to make it more palatable.

10 pitted dried apricots
15 pitted dried prunes
1 1/2 cups water
2 medium apples, washed, peeled and quartered
1 cup water (for thinning)

• In a saucepan, cover dried apricots and prunes with water; bring to a boil. Reduce heat and simmer, partially covered, for 15 minutes.
• Add apples and stir; continue to simmer for another 10 minutes. Remove from heat.
• In blender or food processor, purée mixture (adding more water if necessary) until smooth.
• Pour into ice cube trays and freeze.

Yield: 8 to 10 cubes

DOWN UNDER FRUIT SALAD

1/3 banana, washed and skin removed
1 slice of papaya, washed, skin and seeds removed
1/4 kiwi fruit, washed and skin removed
1 tbsp unsweetened apple juice (approx)

• In bowl, mash banana and papaya with fork. Strain kiwi through fine sieve to remove seeds; mix with banana and papaya.
• Mix fruit with apple juice as needed. Serve immediately, before banana turns brown.

Yield: 1 serving

OKANAGAN SUMMER SALAD

1/4 peach, washed, pit and skin removed (See How to Remove Skin, page 31)

1/4 pear, washed, cored and skin removed

1/2 banana, washed and skin removed

1 tbsp breast milk or formula (approx)

• In small bowl, mash peach, pear and banana with a fork. Add 1 tbsp of milk and mix thoroughly. If mixture seems too thick, add more milk as needed.

Yield: 1 serving

FROM SEVEN MONTHS

BABY'S BACKED UP!

There is a wide range of normal bowel patterns for infants and toddlers, from several daily bowel movements to only one bowel movement every few days. A slowing of the normal pattern for your baby does not necessarily indicate constipation. Grunting, groaning and a red face are all normal displays during stooling and are not an expression of pain. True constipation, on the other hand, is the passing of very hard, painful stools (associated with crying) and is quite rare in infancy. Weaning from breast milk to formula, and changing brands or type of formula are the most common reasons for an alteration in the nature or frequency of stool. Often, a change in the bowel pattern causes more concern for the parent than it does for the baby. Unlike an adult, baby is not aware or distressed by the infrequency of bowel movements. A temporary increase of fiber in the diet will likely alleviate it; try Dried Fruit Purée (recipe, page 55). Contact your doctor if your baby has symptoms of true constipation or if you notice blood in the stool or fever. Don't administer a medicinal laxative to your infant; these can be harmful if used without a doctor's supervision.

PROCEED WITH CAUTION

The following foods should be delayed for various reasons:

SAFE PREPARATION OF FIRST FOODS

FOOD	RECOMMENDATIONS FOR SERVING
Grapes, Raw carrots, Weiners, Sausages, Cherry tomatoes	To prevent choking, serve finely sliced lengthways. Do not serve in circular pieces.
Honey	Do not serve until I year of age to avoid the risk of botulism. Honey may contain botulism spores which cannot be killed by the immature gastrointestinal tract.
Whole milk	Do not serve until I2 months of age. Small amounts in dairy products such as yogurt and cheese may be introduced at 8 months.
Skim, I% and 2% milk	Do not serve until at least 2 years of age, after consultation with your doctor.
Egg white	To avoid possibility of food allergy, do not serve until I year of age.
Egg yolk	May be served, well cooked, at 9 months of age.
Popcorn, Hard candies, Chewing gum, Nuts, Olives, Raw carrots, Raisins	To prevent choking, avoid until 4 years of age. In the case of nuts, there is also the risk of allergy.
Peanut butter, Shellfish	Do not serve until I8 months to avoid possibility of food allergy.

VEGETABLES

Although your baby may seem eager to chew and quite often the first tooth will have appeared by 6 months, it is necessary to cook all vegetables. However, as the teeth appear, your baby will enjoy eating slightly firmer vegetables; therefore you can cut down on cooking time. This also helps to preserve the food's vitamin content and color, making the meal more aesthetically appealing to baby.

SKINNED SEEDED TOMATOES

Some of the recipes in this book will require tomatoes that have been skinned and seeded. To prepare, plunge tomatoes in a saucepan of boiling water for 30 seconds. Remove from water with slotted spoon; allow to cool. Slit skin with a knife and peel. Cut tomato into quarters; remove seeds.

HEAT 'EM UP

Kids and grown-ups alike love tomatoes for their fresh taste and versatility. They are rich in vitamin C and B-complex, iron and potassium. They also contain important substances known as carotenoids, namely beta-carotene and lycopene. Lycopene gives tomatoes and other foods, such as watermelon and pink grapefruit, their red color, and it acts as a potent antioxidant. Scientists believe that antioxidants neutralize harmful substances known as "free radicals." Research into the antioxidant properties of lycopene suggests it lowers the risk of heart disease and prostate cancer. In fact, in studies, eating 10 or more servings a week of tomato products reduced the risk of prostate cancer by 34 percent. The availability of lycopene is even richer if tomatoes are heated.

TOMATO SAUCE

Many of the following recipes will require a cube of tomato sauce. This simple recipe can form the basis of a delicious pasta sauce for the whole family. Just add garlic, salt and pepper to taste.

1/2 onion, finely diced
I tbsp olive oil
I can (I4 oz) diced tomatoes
2 tbsp tomato paste
I/4 cup water
I/3 cup chopped fresh basil

• In frying pan, heat olive oil over low heat; sauté onion until translucent.
• Add tomatoes, tomato paste and water; bring to a boil.
• Turn down heat, and add basil; simmer, partially covered, for 30 minutes, stirring occasionally.
• Pour into ice cube trays and freeze.

Yield: 10 cubes

VICHYSSOISE

2 large potatoes, washed, peeled and cut in cubes
I I/2 leeks, trimmed, washed thoroughly (sections separated) and sliced
2 cups Salt-Free Chicken Stock (approx) (recipe, page 66)
I/4 cup chopped fresh parsley (optional)

• In large saucepan, pour chicken stock over leeks and potatoes, ensuring there is enough stock to cover the vegetables. Bring to a rapid boil. Reduce heat and simmer, partially covered, until tender, 30 minutes, stirring occasionally.
• Remove from heat, add parsley (if using) and stir.
• With a slotted spoon remove vegetables and place in blender or food processor; set leftover stock aside.
• Purée, adding leftover stock as needed, until desired consistency is reached.
• Pour into ice cube trays and freeze.

Yield: 20 to 22 cubes

TEETHING

At approximately 6 to 7 months of age most babies will cut their first tooth. However, some babies are born with teeth and some do not cut their first tooth until over I year of age. Teething may cause drooling, irritability, increased bowel movements and a reluctance to eat solid foods. Teething does *not* cause fever. For babies 3 months or younger, immediately contact your doctor in the event of fever of 100.4°F or greater. To alleviate symptoms of teething, offer your baby something firm to chew on, such as a chilled teething ring. To prevent a painful rash from drooling, use petroleum jelly as a barrier. Offer soft foods but do not force meals, and increase the number of breast milk or formula feedings to alleviate hunger. For continued teething discomfort, use pain-relieving medicine as advised by your doctor. Teeth cleaning should begin with the appearance of the first tooth and should take place twice a day, as well as after sweeter foods such as dried fruit. Start teeth cleaning using a damp washcloth, and switch to a baby toothbrush with a 1/2 pea-size quantity of toothpaste as more teeth appear.

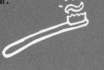

TIME OF ERUPTION OF PRIMARY TEETH

TOOTH TYPE	MONTHS	
	UPPER	LOWER
Front teeth	6 +/- 2	7 +/- 2
Front side teeth	9 +/- 2	7 +/- 2
First molars	14 +/- 4	12 +/- 4
Canines	18 +/- 2	16 +/- 2
Second molars	24 +/- 4	20 +/- 4

VEGETABLE STEW

4 cups Vegetable Stock (not
    optional) (recipe, page 41)

2 carrots, washed, trimmed,
    peeled and sliced

1 parsnip, washed, trimmed,
    peeled and sliced

2 stalks celery, washed, trimmed
    and sliced

1 potato, washed, peeled and cut
    in cubes

1 zucchini, washed, trimmed and
    sliced

1 cup broccoli, washed and cut in
    florets

1/2 leek, trimmed, separated sec-
    tions carefully washed and
    sliced

1/4 cup chopped fresh parsley
    (optional)

• In large saucepan, combine
stock and 7 vegetables. Bring to
a boil. Reduce heat and simmer,
partially covered, for 30 minutes, stirring occasionally.

• Add parsley (if using) and
continue to simmer for another
5 minutes. If there seems to be
too much liquid, remove the
lid for the last 5 to 10 minutes
of cooking time. This will allow
the liquid to evaporate and the
flavors to concentrate.

• Once stew is thick, pour contents through a strainer, separating vegetables from stock;
set stock aside.

• In blender or food processor,
purée vegetables to desired
consistency. Over low heat,
slowly mix vegetables and stock
together, and continue to simmer for another 5 to 10 minutes.
When done, stew should be the
consistency of a thick soup.

• Pour into ice cube trays and
freeze.

Yield: 26 cubes

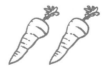

BROWN RICE AND VEGETABLES

2 cups Salt-Free Chicken Stock
(recipe, page 66)
I cup broccoli florets, washed
2 carrots, washed, peeled and cut
in sticks
I/3 cup whole-grain brown rice

• In saucepan, bring stock to boil. Add broccoli and carrots; reduce heat and simmer with lid on to prevent evaporation of stock.
• Once tender, drain vegetables; save stock. (Cooking the vegetables in stock preserves nutrients that would otherwise be lost.)
• Pour stock back into saucepan; add rice.
• Bring to a boil, stir once and reduce heat. Cover and simmer for 50 minutes. Remove from heat and allow to stand for 10 minutes.

• In blender or food processor, purée rice, excess stock and vegetables to desired consistency.
• Pour into ice cube trays and freeze.

Yield: 12 to 14 cubes

RATATOUILLE

This dish is also tasty served with cheese (after 8 months). To prepare, defrost 2 cubes and mix in a saucepan over low heat with 1 tbsp of grated mozzarella cheese.

I can (I4 oz) chopped tomatoes
I cup water
I potato, washed, peeled and cut
in cubes
I cup broccoli florets, washed
I zucchini, washed, trimmed and
sliced
I red pepper, washed, peeled
with potato peeler and diced
I0 green beans, washed, trimmed,
stringy bits removed and
diced
I/3 cup chopped fresh basil
(optional)

• In large saucepan, mix tomatoes and water; add vegetables and bring to a boil. Reduce heat and simmer partially covered for 30 minutes, stirring occasionally. When done, ratatouille should be the consistency of a thick stew. If there is too much liquid, remove the lid for the last 5 to 10 minutes of cooking time. (This allows the flavors to concentrate and the liquid to evaporate.)

• Remove from heat, add basil (if using) and stir.

• With a slotted spoon, remove vegetables and place in blender or food processor. Set leftover cooking juices aside. Purée, adding juices as needed.

• Pour into ice cube trays and freeze.

Yield: 20 to 22 cubes

BROCCOLI AND SWEET POTATO PURÉE

2 sweet potatoes, washed,
   peeled and blemishes
   removed
1 1/2 cups broccoli florets, washed

• Cut sweet potatoes into cubes.

• In saucepan of water, simmer potatoes until tender, 20 to 30 minutes. Remove from water; set leftover cooking water aside.

• Using steamer, steam broccoli over boiling water for 10 minutes.

• In blender or food processor, purée broccoli and potatoes. Add leftover cooking water to achieve desired consistency.

• Pour into ice cube trays and freeze.

Yield: 14 to 16 cubes

SALMONELLA

Salmonella is a bacterial infection of the gastrointestinal tract that affects both children and adults, but, most commonly, infants between 2 and 6 months of age. Sources of infection can be contaminated water, poultry, beef, eggs and milk. It may also be transmitted by infected household pets or other persons. The incubation period is 6 to 72 hours. There is usually an abrupt onset of diarrhea (which may contain blood), vomiting and fever, which may last 2 to 5 days. Symptoms may become severe, particularly in young infants. It is important to contact your doctor if you suspect salmonella. There is usually no antibiotic treatment necessary, but your baby must be monitored to prevent dehydration.

It is very important to prevent contamination of food and utensils by carefully cleaning all surfaces, utensils and refrigerator shelves that have come in contact with raw or partially cooked meat. All meat and eggs should be well cooked before serving, and never serve unpasteurized milk or unpasteurized apple juice. Unlike adults, infants and children have an additional risk of infection from contact with contaminated soil or debris left by pets or shoes. Data suggests this contamination plays an even greater role in infection of children than does contaminated food. To minimize this risk, remove shoes indoors and keep floors clean.

SALT-FREE CHICKEN STOCK

By 7 months, chicken stock, which can easily be made in bulk and frozen, can be used to thin out purées. However, if you do not have the time to make stock, do not let this stop you from preparing homemade chicken for your baby. Many specialty stores now carry salt-free chicken stock. (Avoid using commercial chicken stocks, as they are often high in added salt.) Leftover poaching water can be substituted with adequate results. Stock is best, however, as it serves to enhance flavor and contains calcium that is leached from the chicken bones during cooking.

For this recipe, chicken wings are an economical choice, but any cut will do. A leftover carcass makes a good substitute as well.

3 carrots, washed, peeled and
    sliced

3 stalks celery (including leaves),
    washed and sliced

I onion, cut in chunks

I parsnip, washed, peeled and
    sliced

I sprig fresh rosemary

I bay leaf

6 peppercorns

5 chicken wings

10 cups water

• In large pot, combine vegetables, herbs and chicken. Cover with water and bring to a boil. Turn down heat and simmer, partially covered, until chicken and vegetables release their flavor, 3 to 4 hours.

• Strain the mixture into bowl or pitcher; discard both chicken and vegetables.

• Pour unused stock into ice cube trays and freeze.

Yield: 32 cubes

BABY CHICKEN

2 carrots, washed, peeled and
    sliced
I parsnip, washed, peeled and
    sliced
I/2 Poached Chicken Breast
    (recipe, page 48)
I/4 cup Salt-Free Chicken Stock (2
    to 3 cubes) (recipe, page 66)
or
leftover poaching water

• In steamer, steam carrots and parsnip over boiling water until tender, about 10 minutes.
• In blender or food processor, purée chicken, vegetables and stock to achieve desired consistency. If purée seems too thick, add either extra chicken stock or leftover poaching water.
• *Tip:* For a sweeter version try adding unsweetened apple juice instead of stock.
• Pour into ice cube trays and freeze.

Yield: 10 to 12 cubes

CHICKEN AND WINTER VEGETABLES

I/2 potato, washed, peeled and
    cut in cubes
I carrot, washed, peeled and
    sliced
I cup broccoli florets
I/2 Poached Chicken Breast
    (recipe, page 48)
I/4 cup Salt-Free Chicken Stock (2
    to 3 cubes) (recipe, page 66)
or
leftover poaching water

• In saucepan of boiling water, cook potato for 20 minutes.
• Using steamer, cook carrot and broccoli over boiling water until tender, about 10 minutes.
• In blender or food processor, purée vegetables and chicken, slowly adding chicken stock to achieve desired consistency.
• Pour into ice cube trays and freeze.

Yield: 10 to 12 cubes

SICILIAN CHICKEN

This dish can also be served with cheese (after age 8 months). To prepare, defrost 3 cubes and mix in saucepan over low heat with 1 tbsp of grated Cheddar cheese.

1/4 onion, finely diced

1 tbsp olive oil

2 tomatoes, washed, skinned and
    seeded (recipe, page 60)

1 tbsp chopped fresh parsley
    (optional)

1/2 Poached Chicken Breast
    (recipe, page 48)

1 baked potato, skin removed,
    chopped

• In frying pan, heat olive oil over low heat; sauté onion until translucent.

• Add tomatoes and parsley (if using); continue to sauté for another 10 minutes.

• In blender or food processor, purée tomatoes, chicken and potato to achieve desired consistency.

• Pour into ice cube trays and freeze.

Yield: 10 to 12 cubes

CHICKEN AND BUTTERNUT SQUASH PUREÉ

1 butternut squash, washed and
    ends removed
1/2 Poached Chicken Breast
    (recipe, page 48)
1/4 cup Salt-Free Chicken Stock
    (2 to 3 cubes) (recipe, page 66)
or
leftover poaching water

• Peel squash, cut in half, remove seeds and cut in cubes.
• In steamer, cook squash over boiling water until tender, about 10 to 12 minutes.
•In blender or food processor, purée squash and chicken, adding stock as necessary to achieve desired consistency.
• Pour into ice cube trays and freeze.

Yield: 12 cubes

THANKSGIVING DINNER

1 medium sweet potato, washed,
    peeled and cubed
1/2 Poached Chicken (or Turkey)
    Breast (recipe, page 48)
1/3 cup Salt-Free Chicken Stock
    (3 to 4 cubes) (recipe, page 66)
or
 leftover poaching water

• In saucepan of boiling water, cook sweet potato until tender, 20 to 30 minutes; drain.
• Chop turkey. In blender or food processor, purée turkey, sweet potato and stock. If purée seems too thick, add either extra stock or leftover poaching water to achieve desired consistency.
• Pour into ice cube trays and freeze.

Yield 12 to 14 cubes

PASTA

Most babies love pasta. And the best part is, it's good for them. It is an excellent source of both B vitamins and complex carbohydrates. Complex carbohydrates provide a sustained source of energy that will last throughout the day. Tiny pastines, traditionally used in soups, do not need to be puréed. Larger shapes such as penne or rotini can be served to older babies as finger food. Many of the following recipes can be made in bulk, then puréed and frozen.

To cook dried pasta, place it in boiling, lightly salted water. Add a dash of oil and stir immediately to prevent pasta from sticking. For younger babies, cook 1 minute longer than recommended on the package. Once cooked, drain and rinse pasta under cool water. This rinses off both salt and starch, preventing the pasta from sticking.

Pasta is a wheat product and should not be eaten by babies diagnosed with wheat allergy or gluten intolerance. Please note, however, that gluten and wheat-free pastas are now readily available at most grocery stores and these pastas can be substituted in the following recipes.

MINESTRONE

1 tbsp olive oil

1/4 onion, diced

1 zucchini, washed, trimmed and
   sliced

1 can (14 oz) chopped tomatoes

2 cups Salt-Free Chicken Stock
   (recipe, page 66)

1 1/2 cups broccoli florets, washed

2 carrots, washed, peeled and
   sliced

1/2 cup canned chick-peas,
   drained and rinsed

1/2 cup macaroni

1 handful spinach, washed and
   stalks removed

1/4 cup chopped fresh basil
   (optional)

• In large pot, heat oil over medium heat; sauté onion until translucent, about 5 minutes. Add both zucchini and tomatoes; sauté for another 20 minutes. Stir occasionally.

• Add chicken stock, broccoli, carrots, chick-peas and pasta; bring to a boil. Reduce heat and simmer, partially covered, for 20 minutes.

• Add spinach and basil (if using); continue to simmer for another 10 minutes. The consistency should be that of a thick stew. If there is too much liquid, remove lid for last 5 to 10 minutes of cooking.

• With a slotted spoon, place vegetables, pasta and chick-peas in blender or food processor. Set leftover cooking juices aside.

• Purée, adding leftover juices as needed to achieve desired consistency.

• Pour into ice cube trays and freeze.

Yield: 18 to 20 cubes

CHICKEN NOODLE STEW

1/2 chicken breast, cut in cubes

1 sprig fresh tarragon (optional)

2 cups water

1/3 cup macaroni

1 stalk celery, washed, trimmed and sliced

2 carrots, washed, peeled and sliced

1/4 onion, cut in half

1 potato, washed, peeled and cut in cubes

1/4 cup chopped fresh parsley (optional)

• In large pot, place chicken and tarragon (if using) in water and bring to a boil.

• Add pasta, celery, carrots, onion and potato; reduce heat and simmer, partially covered, until vegetables are tender, about 25 minutes. Stir occasionally. The consistency should be that of a thick stew. If there is too much liquid, remove lid for last 5 to 10 minutes of cooking.

• Remove from heat. Add parsley (if using) and stir.

• Using a slotted spoon, place vegetables, pasta and chicken in blender or food processor. Set leftover cooking juices aside.

• Purée, adding juices as needed to achieve desired consistency.

• Pour into ice cube trays and freeze.

Yield: 18 to 20 cubes

VEGETABLE PRIMAVERA

This recipe can also be served with cheese (after age 8 months). Defrost 3 cubes and mix in a saucepan over low heat with 1 tbsp of grated Cheddar cheese.

I tbsp olive oil

1/4 onion, diced

I zucchini, washed, trimmed and
   sliced

I sweet red pepper, washed,
   peeled with potato peeler
   and diced

I yellow pepper, washed, peeled
   and diced

I can (14 oz) tomatoes, packed in
   their own juice

I 1/2 cups broccoli florets, washed

1/4 cup water

1/3 cup chopped fresh basil
   (optional)

I cup (8 oz) dried pasta, cooked

• In frying pan, heat oil over medium heat; sauté onion until translucent, about 5 minutes. Add zucchini and peppers; continue to sauté, stirring occasionally, for 20 minutes.

• Stir in tomatoes, broccoli and water; simmer, partially covered, until broccoli is tender, about 20 minutes.

• Remove from heat; stir in basil (if using) and cooked pasta.

• Empty mixture into blender or food processor and purée.

• Pour into ice cube trays and freeze.

Yield: 22 to 24 cubes

WHAT ARE NURSING CARIES?

Nursing caries or "nursing bottle syndrome" refers to the damaging effects of continuous bottle-feeding to the teeth. If teeth are continuously bathed in nutrient-containing liquids such as milk, fruit juice or other sugar-containing drinks there is a continual supply of sugar on which dental bacteria proliferate and this may cause cavities. This is most likely to occur in a baby over 12 months old who is given a bottle for sleep or as a pacifier. When the baby falls asleep liquid may pool in the mouth and coat the teeth. A baby who discards the bottle prior to falling asleep is at much less risk than one who falls asleep with the bottle in her mouth. Beware of propping up the bottle so baby can self-feed, which can contribute to dental caries and cause choking. Liquids other than breast milk should be given in a cup by 12 months of age, and try to switch to water at bedtime if a bottle is necessary to fall asleep. Tooth brushing should begin with the appearance of the first tooth and occur twice a day, using a baby toothbrush with a 1/2 pea-size amount of toothpaste.

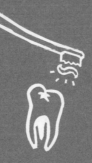

RED MEAT

In an effort to minimize the risk of heart disease and stroke, many people now avoid red meat. Others believe that reduced intake of carbohydrates and increased intake of lean meats, including red meat, actually reduces obesity and heart disease in adults. Studies show that cholesterol and animal fat intake during infancy does not contribute to heart disease later in life. Further, iron deficiency is the most common nutritional problem among children and may have serious health consequences. Thus, as red meat is the richest source of iron available, its consumption will benefit your baby.

The method of choice for cooking red meat is stewing, as it tenderizes the meat while it cooks.

IRON-DEFICIENCY ANEMIA

Iron is a major component of hemoglobin, which enables red blood cells to transport oxygen throughout the body. Iron deficiency is a common finding among infants, children and teenagers. Risk factors for the development of iron-deficiency anemia include pre-maturity, low birth weight, anemia in the mother during pregnancy, too early introduction of cow's milk or solid foods, low meat intake, breastfeeding beyond 6 months without other sources of iron, infant formula not supplemented with iron, and some unusual dietary practices.

During the rapid growth period in the first year of life, infants almost triple their blood volume, and their requirement for iron increases from 4 mg per day to 7 mg per day. These requirements are higher for premature infants. If iron needs are not met, infants may become deficient, which leads to poor weight gain, recurrent illness, poor appetite, gastrointestinal problems, irritability, decreased attention span and decreased physical activity. If the deficiency persists it is possible that cognitive development may be impaired. If iron deficiency is suspected, a blood test can confirm the diagnosis.

To maintain your baby's adequate iron intake be sure her diet includes a wide variety of iron-rich foods such as iron-fortified baby cereals, poultry, red meat, broccoli, spinach and legumes. Continue iron-fortified baby cereals throughout the first two years by mixing with other foods and serving often. The amount of iron in infant formula and supplements is often much higher than the recommended daily intake because the amount of iron actually absorbed by the body is quite small. To enhance absorption, serve iron-rich foods with foods high in vitamin C such as tomatoes, baked potato and citrus fruits.

MAMA'S HOMEMADE BEEF STEW

8 cubes stewing beef

2 cups water

2 carrots, washed, trimmed, peeled and sliced

I potato, washed, peeled and cut in cubes

1/4 onion, cut in half

2 celery stalks, washed, trimmed and sliced

2 chopped fresh sage leaves (optional)

2 sprigs fresh parsley (optional)

• In large pot, bring beef and water to a boil. Add carrots, potato, onion, celery and herbs (if using). Reduce heat and simmer, partially covered, until meat is thoroughly cooked and vegetables are tender, about 25 to 30 minutes. Stir occasionally. The consistency should be that of a thick stew. If there is too much liquid, remove lid for last 5 to 10 minutes of cooking. (This enables the water to evaporate and the flavors to concentrate.)

• With a slotted spoon, place meat and vegetables in blender or food processor. Set leftover cooking juices aside. Purée, adding juices as needed to achieve desired consistency.

• Pour into ice cube trays and freeze.

Yield: 18 to 20 cubes

MAXWELL'S MINTED LAMB

I cup water

I can (14 oz) diced tomatoes

8 cubes stewing lamb

I potato, washed, peeled and cut
   in cubes

2 carrots, washed, peeled and
   sliced

2 stalks celery, washed, trimmed
   and sliced

1/4 onion, diced

I tbsp chopped fresh mint
   (optional)

• In saucepan, mix water with tomatoes and add lamb. Bring to a boil.

• Add vegetables; reduce heat and continue to simmer until they are tender, 25 to 30 minutes. Stir occasionally. The consistency should be that of a thick stew. If you feel there is too much liquid, remove the lid for last 5 to 10 minutes of cooking. (This will allow the water to evaporate and flavors to concentrate.)

• Add mint (if using) and stir.

• With a slotted spoon place lamb and vegetables in blender or food processor. Set leftover cooking juices aside.

• Purée, adding juices as needed to achieve desired consistency.

• Pour into ice cube trays and freeze.

Yield: 18 to 20 cubes

SHEPHERD'S MASH

I tbsp olive oil

1/4 onion, diced

I can (14 oz) diced tomatoes

I tbsp chopped fresh parsley
   (optional)

I carrot, washed, peeled and sliced

I clove garlic, mashed (optional)

8 cubes stewing beef

1/4 cup water

2 medium potatoes, washed,
   peeled and cut in cubes

• In saucepan, heat oil over medium heat; sauté onion until translucent, about 5 minutes. Stir in tomatoes, parsley, carrot and garlic (if using); continue to sauté for another 5 minutes.

• Add beef and water; bring to a boil. Reduce heat and simmer, partially covered, until meat is thoroughly cooked, 25 to 30 minutes. Stir occasionally.

• Meanwhile, in saucepan of boiling salted water cook potatoes until tender; drain.

• In blender or food processor, purée meat mixture and potatoes until desired consistency is reached. Pour into ice cube trays and freeze.

Yield: 16 to 18 cubes

PORK AND APPLE PURÉE

8 cubes stewing pork
I cup water
4 apples, washed, peeled, cored
    and sectioned

• In saucepan, bring pork and water to a boil. Reduce heat and simmer, partially covered, until pork is thoroughly cooked, 25 to 30 minutes. Set aside and save stewing water.

• In steamer, steam apples over boiling water for 10 minutes.

• In blender or food processor, purée apples and pork to achieve desired consistency. (For younger babies it may be necessary to add leftover stewing water to thin out the purée.) When adding liquid, start with 1 tbsp at a time.

• Pour into ice cube trays and freeze.

Yield: 12 cubes

EASY BEEF HASH

I/2 lb ground beef
I cup canned diced tomatoes
I potato, washed and baked

• Brown beef in a nonstick frying pan for 5 minutes, until no longer pink. Add tomatoes and continue to sauté for another 10 minutes, stirring occasionally.

• Meanwhile, cut potato in half, scoop out flesh and mash with a fork. Add potato to pan; continue to sauté for 10 minutes.

• Pour into ice cube trays and freeze.

• *Tip:* For very young babies you may choose to purée in a food processor before freezing.

Yield: 12 to 14 cubes

MIDDLE-EASTERN
BEEF STEW

2 tbsp olive oil

1/4 onion, diced

I tsp freshly grated ginger
(optional)

I tsp ground cumin (optional)

1/2 medium eggplant, washed,
peeled and diced

I can (I9 oz) chick-peas, drained
and rinsed

8 cubes stewing beef

I carrot, washed, peeled and sliced

2 cups water

1/4 cup chopped fresh parsley
(optional)

• In saucepan, heat oil over medium heat; sauté onion and ginger for 5 minutes. Add cumin, eggplant and chick-peas; continue to sauté for another 20 minutes.

• Add beef, carrot and water; stir. Bring to a boil. Reduce heat and simmer, partially covered, until meat is cooked, 25 to 30 minutes. Stir occasionally. The consistency should be that of a thick stew. If you feel there is too much liquid, remove the lid for last 5 to 10 minutes of cooking. (This will allow the water to evaporate and flavors to concentrate.)

• Remove from heat. Add parsley (if using) and stir.

• With a slotted spoon, place beef, vegetables and chick-peas in blender or food processor. Set leftover cooking juices aside. Purée, adding juices as needed to achieve desired consistency.

• Pour into ice cube trays and freeze.

Yield: 16 to 18 cubes

SAMPLE WEEKLY MEAL PLANNER: FROM SEVEN TO EIGHT MONTHS

WEEK I

DAY I

Breakfast	Breast or Bottle, Florida Breakfast
Mid-A.M. Snack	Breast or Bottle
Lunch	Pork and Apple Purée
Mid-P.M. Snack	Breast or Bottle
Dinner	Vichyssoise, Mashed Banana
Before Bed	Breast or Bottle

DAY 2

Breakfast	Breast or Bottle, Single-Grain Cereal (Oats) Mashed Banana
Mid-A.M. Snack	Breast or Bottle
Lunch	Chicken Apple Delight
Mid-P.M. Snack	Breast or Bottle
Dinner	Vegetable Stew
Before Bed	Breast or Bottle

DAY 3

Breakfast	Breast or Bottle, Single-Grain Cereal (Wheat) and Apple Purée
Mid-A.M. Snack	Breast or Bottle
Lunch	Chicken Noodle Stew, Mashed Pear
Mid-P.M. Snack	Breast or Bottle
Dinner	Mashed Avocado and Banana
Before Bed	Breast or Bottle

DAY 4

Breakfast	Breast or Bottle, Single-Grain Cereal (Rice) and Mashed Banana
Mid-A.M. Snack	Breast or Bottle
Lunch	Ratatouille, Mashed Avocado
Mid-P.M. Snack	Breast or Bottle
Dinner	Shepherd's Mash and Pear Purée
Before Bed	Breast or Bottle

DAY 5

Breakfast	Breast or Bottle, Mixed-Grain Cereal and Mashed Banana
Mid-A.M. Snack	Breast or Bottle
Lunch	Thanksgiving Dinner
Mid-P.M. Snack	Breast or Bottle
Dinner	Vegetable Primavera, Melon
Before Bed	Breast or Bottle

Baby may also wake for additional feeds during the night.

You may mix any of the purées with baby cereal for palatability and increased iron.

SAMPLE WEEKLY MEAL PLANNER: FROM SEVEN TO EIGHT MONTHS

WEEK 1 continued

DAY 6	
Breakfast	Breast or Bottle, Single-Grain Cereal (Oats) and Pear Purée
Mid-A.M. Snack	Breast or Bottle
Lunch	Baby Bunny's Purée, Apple Purée
Mid PM Snack	Breast or Bottle
Dinner	Chicken and Winter Vegetables
Before Bed	Breast or Bottle

DAY 7	
Breakfast	Breast or Bottle, Single-Grain Cereal (Wheat) and Apple Purée
Mid-A.M. Snack	Breast or Bottle
Lunch	Easy Beef Hash, Mashed Banana
Mid-P.M. Snack	Breast or Bottle
Dinner	Broccoli Watercress and Potato Purée
Before Bed	Breast or Bottle

SAMPLE WEEKLY MEAL PLANNER: FROM SEVEN TO EIGHT MONTHS

WEEK 2

DAY 1	
Breakfast	Breast or Bottle, Single-Grain Cereal (Oats) and Pear Purée
Mid-A.M. Snack	Breast or Bottle
Lunch	Mama's Homemade Beef Stew
Mid PM Snack	Breast or Bottle
Dinner	Mashed Avocado and Papaya
Before Bed	Breast or Bottle

DAY 2	
Breakfast	Breast or Bottle, Single-Grain Cereal (Oats) and Mashed Papaya
Mid-A.M. Snack	Breast or Bottle
Lunch	Vegetable Stew and Whole-Wheat Toast Strips
Mid-P.M. Snack	Breast or Bottle
Dinner	Baby Chicken and Mashed Banana
Before Bed	Breast or Bottle

WEEK 2 continued

DAY 3

Breakfast	Breast or Bottle, Fruit Cereal
Mid-A.M. Snack	Breast or Bottle
Lunch	Sicilian Chicken
Mid-P.M. Snack	Breast or Bottle
Dinner	Broccoli Watercress and Potato
Before Bed	Breast or Bottle

DAY 4

Breakfast	Breast or Bottle, Florida Breakfast
Mid-A.M. Snack	Breast or Bottle
Lunch	Baby Chicken
Mid-P.M. Snack	Breast or Bottle
Dinner	Minestrone, Mashed Banana
Before Bed	Breast or Bottle

DAY 5

Breakfast	Breast or Bottle, Single-Grain Cereal (Rice)
Mid-A.M. Snack	Breast or Bottle
Lunch	Vegetable Primavera
Mid-P.M. Snack	Breast or Bottle
Dinner	Vichyssoise, Mashed Avocado
Before Bed	Breast or Bottle

DAY 6

Breakfast	Breast or Bottle, Single-Grain Cereal (Wheat) and Mashed Pear
Mid-A.M. Snack	Breast or Bottle
Lunch	Baby Bunny's Purée and Whole-Wheat Toast Strips
Mid-P.M. Snack	Breast or Bottle
Dinner	Shepherd's Mash
Before Bed	Breast or Bottle

DAY 7

Breakfast	Breast or Bottle, Single-Grain Cereal (Barley) and Apple Purée
Mid-A.M. Snack	Breast or Bottle
Lunch	Okanagan Summer Chicken
Mid-P.M. Snack	Breast or Bottle
Dinner	Brown Rice and Vegetables
Before Bed	Breast or Bottle

Baby may also wake for additional feeds during the night.

You may mix any of the purées with baby cereal for palatability and increased iron.

From Eight Months

By 8 months of age your baby will enjoy eating slightly lumpier textures. Instead of puréeing the foods, try mashing them with a fork or using a blender or food processor in short pulses to aid in mixing or chopping. This is the time to introduce finger foods as he now has the dexterity to pick up small pieces of food. Although not likely to become proficient with a spoon until at least 12 months, he should be encouraged in his attempts to self-feed. With each little triumph his confidence will grow.

By 10 months of age some babies reject being spoon-fed altogether, while others continue for many months. If this happens and your baby is not yet proficient with a spoon, don't despair—healthy meals can be made up entirely of finger foods (see Finger Food, page 125).

FRUIT

At 8 months your baby may enjoy a wider variety of fresh, soft fruits. Fruits may no longer need to be mashed and can be served in small pieces. Indulge your baby's need for independence by offering a bowl of interesting fruits from which he can choose, and which he can serve himself.

This is a sensible time to introduce calcium-rich dairy products, such as yogurt and cheese. (Cow's milk for drinking should be postponed until 12 months.) These recommendations will be different if there is a family history of true cow's milk allergy. (Please see Adverse Reactions and Allergies, page 25, and consult your physician.) Remember to always serve whole-fat dairy products (for example, 3.25% milk; above 3% yogurt) to your baby. Avoid adult soy beverages until 2 years as the fat content is too low for babies, equivalent to 2% milk.

Tip: fresh fruit combined with yogurt makes delicious fruit smoothies.

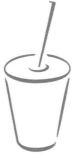

CARIBBEAN-STYLE COTTAGE CHEESE

Cottage cheese mixes well with other fruits. Try it with either grated apple or mashed banana.

2 slices papaya, washed and skin
    removed
1/3 cup cottage cheese

• In small bowl, mash papaya with fork. Mix cottage cheese with fruit, and serve.

Yield: 1 serving

FIT FOR LIFE

Life expectancy in many nations consistently exceeds predicted forecasts. In the 1920s life expectancy averaged age 65. In 1990 it was 85. Now it is believed that a baby girl born in Japan or France (countries with the highest life expectancy) has a 50-percent chance of living to 100! With the prospect of this longevity, it is important to equip children with strong skeletons. Osteoporosis is a disease that causes a stooped spine and weak, easily broken bones. Symptoms usually begin after 50 but prevention begins in infancy with the development of strong bones from adequate calcium intake. Plenty of calcium, exercise and vitamin D will help to reduce the risk of osteoporosis. Dairy is the best source of calcium, but adequate intake may be achieved with alternative sources.

DRIED FRUIT YOGURT

1 cube Dried Fruit Purée (recipe,
   page 57)
1/3 cup high-fat (above 3%) plain
   yogurt

Dried fruit purée has a rather
strong flavor, so mixing it with
yogurt makes it more palatable.
Defrost purée. Mix in bowl
with yogurt, and serve at room
temperature.

Yield: 1 serving

HOW TALL WILL BABY GROW?

Since height is partly genetically determined, it is possible to estimate a
child's adult height based on the parents' height. The estimate has a range
of +/- 18 cm (3.15 inches).

FOR A BOY

$$\frac{(\text{Father's height in cm} + \text{Mother's height in cm} + 13)}{2}$$

FOR A GIRL

$$\frac{(\text{Father's height in cm} - 13 + \text{Mother's height in cm})}{2}$$

FRUIT SMOOTHIE

This recipe can be made with either mashed banana or any of your baby's favorite fruit purées.

I cube fruit purée
I/3 cup high-fat (above 3%) plain
    yogurt
I tbsp unsweetened apple juice
    (approx)

• Defrost 1 cube of your baby's favorite fruit purée; mix with yogurt. If the mixture seems too thick, add unsweetened apple juice 1 tbsp at a time.

Yield: 1 serving

TROPICAL SMOOTHIE

I slice mango, washed, skin
    removed
I/3 banana, washed, skin removed
2 tbsp high-fat (above 3%) plain
    yogurt
I tbsp unsweetened apple juice
    (approx)

• In small bowl, mash mango and banana with fork. Using blender or food processor, purée fruit, yogurt and juice. Serve immediately, before the banana turns brown.

Yield: 1 serving

AVOCADO SMOOTHIE

I/3 avocado, washed, pit and skin
    removed
I/3 cup high-fat (above 3%) plain
    yogurt

• In small bowl, mash avocado with fork. Mix with yogurt; serve.

Yield: 1 serving

89

VEGETABLES

Starting a meal with steamed vegetable sticks is a great way to entertain baby while you feed him. At this stage your baby will also enjoy eating steamed vegetables puréed with cheese. When making vegetable-and-cheese mixtures, cutting down on the puréeing time will provide lumpier and more interesting textures for older babies. All cheeses *must* be pasteurized. Cheddar, mozzarella, Edam, and cottage cheese are popular choices.

FLORETS AND CHEESE SAUCE

For older babies, steam florets and serve sauce on the side, as they will enjoy dipping the vegetables into the sauce. Try serving the sauce with different vegetables, such as thinly sliced steamed beans, soft-cooked carrots or quartered cherry tomatoes.

I tbsp butter

I tbsp flour (approx)

I cup breast milk or formula

I 1/2 cups grated, mature Cheddar
    cheese, firmly packed (6 oz)

2 cups broccoli florets, washed

2 cups cauliflower florets,
    washed

• *To prepare cheese sauce:* In saucepan, whisk butter and flour together over medium heat until paste forms. Slowly add 1/2 cup of milk, whisking until lumps disappear. Continue to whisk, while adding cheese and the remaining milk. Stir until cheese melts and sauce thickens to a smooth, creamy texture.

• In steamer, cook florets over boiling water for 10 minutes. In blender or food processor, combine with cheese sauce and purée to achieve desired consistency.

• Pour into ice cube trays and freeze.

Yield: 16 cubes

PEAS, PLEASE

Peas are introduced after age 8 months, as very young babies may find the outer shells difficult to digest. You can use either fresh or frozen peas. Frozen peas are more convenient; however fresh peas are sweeter in flavor and more likely to appeal. As frozen foods should not be refrozen, only fresh peas can be made in bulk. The following recipes are for fresh and frozen peas.

2 cups freshly shelled peas
3 tbsp breast milk or formula
    (approx)

• Using steamer, cook peas over boiling water for 5 minutes.
• In blender or food processor, purée peas, adding milk to achieve desired consistency.
• Pour into ice cube trays and freeze.

Yield: 8 to 10 cubes

FROZEN PEAS

1/2 cup frozen peas
1/2 cup water
1 tbsp breast milk or formula

• In saucepan, combine frozen peas and water; bring to a boil. Reduce heat and cook until peas are tender, 2 to 3 minutes; drain.
• Either mash peas and milk together with a fork, or use blender or food processor to purée to achieve desired consistency.

Yield: 1 serving

WHAT ABOUT SALT?

Sodium is an essential dietary nutrient that plays an important role in metabolism and maintenance of blood pressure.

Sodium occurs naturally in many foods, including cow's milk, human milk, cheese, vegetables and grain. It also can be added to foods in the form of salt. In adults, an excess of sodium can raise blood pressure and cause significant health problems in later life. As it is not clear what the consequences of excess sodium are for infants, it seems wise not to use added salt when preparing baby food. For older children, moderate use of salt in a few selected foods is acceptable. Most important, parents should consider their habits and model moderate intake so that as the child begins to eat from the family table, she learns not to over-salt.

BROCCOLI SURPRISE

Tomato sauce mixes very well with most vegetables. To make other delicious combinations, follow this recipe substituting your baby's favorite purée for the broccoli.

I cube Tomato Sauce (recipe, page 6I)
2 cubes Broccoli Purée (recipe, page 40)
I tbsp grated Cheddar cheese

• Defrost cubes.
• In saucepan, mix over low heat. Add cheese, stirring occasionally.
• Remove from heat; cool to room temperature.

Yield: 1 serving

SPINACH AND CHEESE

1 potato, washed, peeled and cut
    in cubes
4 handfuls of spinach, washed
    and thick stalks removed
1/3 cup grated Cheddar cheese,
    loosely packed (1.5 oz)
1/2 cup cottage cheese
1/4 cup Vegetable Stock (2 to 3
    cubes) (recipe, page 41)
or
leftover cooking water (optional)

• In saucepan of boiling water, cook potato for 20 minutes; drain, reserving leftover cooking water.
• In steamer, cook spinach for 5 minutes.
• In blender or food processor, purée vegetables and cheese. If mixture seems too thick, add either stock or leftover cooking water as required.
• Pour into ice cube trays and freeze.

Yield: 10 to 12 cubes

QUICK CARROT AND PARSNIP AU GRATIN

3 carrots, washed, peeled and
    sliced
3 parsnips, washed, peeled and
    sliced
1 cup grated Gruyère cheese (4 oz)
1/4 cup Vegetable Stock (2 to 3
    cubes) (recipe, page 41)
or
leftover cooking water (optional)

• In steamer, steam vegetables for 15 minutes.
• In blender or food processor, purée vegetables and cheese. If purée seems too thick, add either stock or leftover cooking water to achieve desired consistency.
• Pour into ice cube trays and freeze.

Yield: 12 to 14 cubes

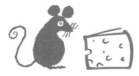

93

BAKED TOMATO AND ZUCCHINI AU GRATIN

This dish makes a quick and satisfying vegetable accompaniment to family meals. Just add salt, pepper and garlic to taste.

2 tbsp olive oil

4 zucchinis, washed, trimmed and
   sliced

10 mushrooms, washed and sliced

4 tomatoes, skinned and seeded,
   diced (recipe, page 60)

1 1/2 cups grated Cheddar cheese
   (6 oz)

1/4 cup grated Parmesan cheese
   (1 oz)

2 tbsp chopped fresh basil
   (optional)

• In large frying pan, heat oil over medium heat; sauté zucchini and mushrooms, stirring occasionally, until zucchini is golden brown, 25 to 30 minutes.

• In ovenproof dish, layer zucchini mixture, tomatoes and Cheddar cheese. Sprinkle with Parmesan cheese and basil (if using).

• Bake in 375°F oven for 30 minutes. Remove from oven and cool.

• In blender or food processor, purée to desired consistency.

• Pour into ice cube trays and freeze.

Yield: 16 cubes

SUPERBABY'S SPINACH PURÉE

4 handfuls of spinach, washed
   and stalks removed
I large potato, washed and baked,
   skin removed
2 tbsp breast milk or formula
   (approx)

• In steamer, steam spinach over boiling water for 5 minutes.
• In blender or food processor, purée potato and spinach, adding milk as needed to achieve desired consistency.
• Pour into ice cube trays and freeze.

Yield: 10 cubes

ROASTED VEGGIE MASH

I potato, washed and peeled
4 small beets, washed and peeled
I carrot, washed, trimmed and
   peeled
I parsnip, washed, trimmed and
   peeled
2 tbsp olive oil
I tbsp butter
2 tbsp breast milk or formula
   (approx)

• Cut potato, beets, carrot and parsnip into cubes. In bowl, toss with olive oil.
• In roasting pan, bake vegetables in 375°F oven for 30 minutes. Flip vegetables and bake until tender, 25 to 30 minutes. Remove from oven to cool.
• For a nice lumpy texture, add butter and milk as needed; mash with potato masher (or if desired, use blender or food processor to purée until smooth).
• Pour into ice cube trays and freeze.

Yield: 12 to 14 cubes

BEANS AND GRAINS

BEANS Beans and lentils are rich in both iron and protein. At this stage your baby will be ready to eat lumpier textures, so, instead of puréeing the beans, try mashing with a fork to preserve texture. Always rinse and drain canned beans and vegetables to remove the salt.

IS IT SAFE TO FEED BABY A VEGETARIAN DIET?

In adults, the health benefits of reducing animal fat intake are well known; however, whether vegetarian diets are healthy for a growing baby remains controversial. It is possible to develop serious vitamin, mineral and fatty acid deficiencies, as the requirement for these nutrients is higher in babies and children than it is in adults. It is known, for example, that the risk of iron deficiency is much higher for those on a vegetarian diet. A strict vegan diet (without dairy or animal products) is not safe for children under 2. Vegetarian parents may benefit from a consultation from a pediatric dietitian to ensure baby's nutrient demands are being met.

TUSCAN TOMATO AND CHICK-PEAS

1/2 onion, diced

1 tbsp olive oil

2 zucchini, washed, trimmed, sliced and diced

1 can (14 oz) chopped tomatoes

1 can (19 oz) chick-peas, rinsed and drained

Pinch cumin (optional)

1/3 cup chopped fresh basil (optional)

• In frying pan, heat oil and sauté onion on low heat until translucent, about 5 minutes. Add zucchini and continue to sauté, stirring occasionally, for 20 minutes.

• Add tomatoes, chick-peas and cumin (if using) and simmer, partially covered, for 30 minutes. Stir occasionally.

• Remove from heat, add basil (if using) and stir. Mash with fork.

• Fill ice cube trays and freeze.

Yield: 16 cubes

NAVY BEANS

1 tbsp olive oil

1/2 onion, diced

1 zucchini, washed, trimmed, sliced and diced

1 sweet red pepper, washed, peeled with potato peeler and diced

1 can (14 oz) chopped tomatoes

1 carrot, washed, peeled, sliced and diced

1 can (19 oz) navy beans, rinsed and drained

1/2 cup chopped fresh basil (optional)

• In frying pan, heat oil over medium heat; sauté onion until translucent, about 5 minutes. Add zucchini and red pepper; continue to sauté for another 15 minutes, stirring occasionally.

• Add tomatoes, carrot and beans to frying pan; simmer, partially covered, for another 30 minutes.

• Remove from heat, add basil (if using) and stir. Mash with fork.

• Fill ice cube trays and freeze.

Yield: 16 cubes

GREEN LENTILS

1 tbsp oil
1/2 onion, diced
1 stalk celery, washed, trimmed
    and sliced
1 clove garlic, crushed (optional)
1 tsp curry powder
1 can (14 oz) diced tomatoes
1 can (19 oz) green lentils, drained
    and rinsed
3 tbsp tomato paste
1/4 cup chopped fresh cilantro or
    basil (optional)

• In frying pan, heat oil over medium heat; sauté onion and celery until onion is translucent, about 5 minutes. Reduce heat; stir in garlic and curry powder. Continue to sauté for another 5 minutes.
• Add tomatoes, lentils and tomato paste; sauté for another 35 minutes.
• Remove from heat and add cilantro or basil (if using). Mix thoroughly. Mash with fork.
• Fill ice cube trays and freeze.

Yield: 16 cubes

CHICK-PEAS AU GRATIN

1/2 onion, diced
1 tbsp olive oil
1 can (14 oz) chopped tomatoes
1/4 cup water
1 can (19 oz) chick-peas, drained
    and rinsed
2 cups broccoli, cut in baby-bite-
    size pieces
1/3 cup grated Cheddar cheese
    (1.5 oz)
1 tbsp chopped fresh basil
    (optional)

• In frying pan, heat oil over medium heat; sauté onion until translucent, about 5 minutes. Add tomatoes, water, chick-peas and broccoli; increase heat and bring to a boil. Reduce heat and simmer, partially covered, 30 minutes. Remove from heat.
• Add cheese and basil (if using), and stir until cheese is thoroughly melted. Mash with fork.
• Fill ice cube trays and freeze.

Yield: 18 to 20 cubes

THE IMPORTANCE OF ZINC

Dietary zinc plays diverse roles in metabolic functions of the body. Growth velocity, immune function, appetite, cognitive function and behavior are all dependent on sufficient zinc levels in the diet. Some diaper rashes may suggest zinc deficiency and will improve by increasing dietary zinc and by applying a diaper cream containing zinc. Adequate levels of zinc are also thought to help protect the body from metal toxicity such as lead poisoning. The best supply of zinc is from animal sources such as meat, eggs (do not offer whole eggs until I year of age) and human milk. Zinc is also available in legumes, potatoes and whole grains but is not as well absorbed as animal sources of zinc. Fortified breakfast cereals and baby cereals are also good sources for infants and children.

NOTE: Couscous is a wheat product and therefore should not be served to babies with wheat allergy or gluten intolerance.

SWEET PEPPER COUSCOUS

I/2 onion, diced

I tbsp olive oil

I sweet red pepper, washed, peeled
   with potato peeler and
   finely diced

I sweet yellow pepper, washed,
   peeled and finely diced

I/4 cup chopped fresh basil
   (optional)

I tsp olive oil

I/2 cup water

I/2 cup couscous

• In frying pan, heat oil over medium heat; sauté onion until translucent, about 5 minutes. Add peppers and continue to sauté for 25 minutes. Stir in basil (if using) and set aside.

• In saucepan, add 1 tsp olive oil to water and bring to a boil. Pour couscous into water, cover with lid and remove from heat. Allow to stand for 5 minutes. Fluff with fork and allow to stand for another 5 minutes. Once couscous is fluffy in consistency, add peppers and mix thoroughly.

• *Tip:* For younger babies you may choose to use a blender or food processor to purée couscous before freezing.

• Fill ice cube trays and freeze.

Yield: 10 cubes

LIZ'S COUSCOUS

1/2 cup diced onion

1 tbsp olive oil

2 zucchinis, washed, trimmed and
   finely diced

1 tsp olive oil

1/2 cup water

1/2 cup couscous

• In frying pan, heat oil over medium heat; sauté onion until translucent, about 5 minutes. Add zucchini and continue to sauté until zucchini is thoroughly cooked, about 25 minutes.

• In saucepan, add 1 tsp olive oil to water and bring to a boil. Pour couscous into water, cover with lid and remove from heat.

Allow to stand for 5 minutes. Fluff with fork and allow to stand for another 5 minutes. Once couscous is fluffy in consistency, add zucchini and mix thoroughly.

• *Tip:* For younger babies, you may choose to use a blender or food processor to purée couscous before freezing.

• Fill ice cube trays and freeze.

Yield: 10 cubes

VEGETABLE BARLEY RISOTTO

This tempting and nutrient-packed dish makes a hearty accompaniment to a family meal. Just add salt and pepper to taste. Barley should not be consumed by babies diagnosed with gluten intolerance.

1 cup barley

2 tbsp olive oil

1/2 onion, diced

1 stalk celery, washed, trimmed
   and finely diced

1 carrot washed, peeled and
   grated using a cheese grater

1/2 bulb fennel, outer layer
removed, sections separated
and washed, finely diced
1 clove garlic, mashed (optional)
3 1/2 cups Salt-Free Chicken
Stock (recipe, page 66)
1 tbsp chopped fresh parsley
(optional)

• Rinse barley and set aside.
• In frying pan, heat oil and sauté vegetables and garlic (if using) over medium heat until vegetables are tender, about 10 minutes.
• Add barley and continue to stir. Add enough stock to cover barley; bring to a boil. Reduce heat and simmer, stirring occasionally, for 30 to 35 minutes. Add stock as needed to keep the barley covered. Once cooked, barley should be tender but firm.
• Add parsley (if using); stir.
• Fill ice cube trays and freeze.
• *Tip:* For younger babies you may choose to use a blender or food processor to purée barley before freezing.

Yield: 16 cubes

HERBAL MEDICATIONS, REMEDIES AND TEAS

The use of herbal products is widespread and increasing in many countries. Parents should consider potential hazards, however—especially for babies, who are more prone to toxicity than adults. Some products may not be subject to stringent manufacturing codes. This can lead to poor standardization; contamination with pesticides, heavy metals and other carcinogenic compounds; adulteration with other pharmaceuticals; and incorrect dosage and labeling. Furthermore, the claims made about some products may be unfounded. There have been many cases of serious electrolyte disturbances and other toxic effects in babies and children given these products. The bottom line: herbal preparations are not recommended for babies.

CHICKEN

By age 8 months babies can eat chicken that is not finely puréed. Pulsing your blender or food processor will aid in mixing and chopping, while retaining some texture.

Baby appetites and sizes vary greatly. Provided your little one is developing normally, you need not be overly concerned about comparing him with other babies. Offer nutritious snacks and meals and be reassured that no healthy baby will starve himself. There is also no correlation between big babies and overweight adults. Please vary recipe quantities according to your baby's appetite.

CHARLIE'S CHEESY CHICKEN

Charlie's Cheesy Chicken combines very well with a variety of vegetable purées. Defrost 2 cubes Cheesy Chicken and 2 cubes broccoli purée. Combine in saucepan over low heat, and serve. Try a variety of other delicious combinations by substituting any of the vegetable purées for the broccoli.

1/2 Poached Chicken Breast
  (recipe, page 48)
1/2 cup cottage cheese
1/3 cup grated Cheddar cheese
  (1.5 oz)
1/4 cup Salt-Free Chicken Stock
  (2 to 3 cubes) (recipe, page 66)
or
leftover poaching water

• In blender or food processor, purée chicken, cottage cheese and Cheddar cheese. Add stock, as needed, to achieve desired consistency.

Yield: 14 cubes

FOOD REFUSAL

Beginning at about 8 months of age it is common for babies to refuse meals. They demonstrate this by shutting the mouth, turning the head or throwing food. Often the refusal occurs even if the baby is hungry and before the meal is even tasted. It is very important that parents recognize that this is a normal developmental stage and it does not represent defiance. It may also signal a desire for independence and the opportunity for baby to feed herself. Giving baby a spoon to hold and encouraging self-feeding attempts may help.

Nevertheless, refusal often persists and can become very frustrating for parents. Resist force-feeding or punishing your baby. Instead increase nutritious snacks to alleviate hunger. This does not set a bad precedent; at this young age, a baby does not understand that refusing at one time leads to snacks at another. Continue to include your baby in family mealtimes but postpone the essential "three square meals" until later in childhood. If your baby has persistent low appetite, discuss the possibility of iron deficiency with your physician.

WHY BOTHER?

Often a well-meaning parent can become discouraged by a baby's continual refusal of food. This is especially true for those who have committed to homemade baby food, investing precious time and energy in preparing nutritious meals, only to be met with refusal and protest. One may ask, why bother? Considering your child will depend on you for proper nutrition and the potential to shape food choices and consequently her health, it is important to persevere. Children who observe your commitment to nutritious eating, even if it requires more time and energy, will likely carry this philosophy with them into adulthood.

CHICKEN CACCIATORE

2 cubes Charlie's Cheesy Chicken
 (recipe, page 102)
I cube Tomato Sauce (recipe,
 page 61)

• Defrost cubes. Heat in saucepan over low heat until warm. Serve.

Yield: 1 serving

BAJA CHICKEN SALAD

2 oz Poached Chicken Breast
 (1/8 of whole) (recipe, page 48)
I slice avocado, washed, skin
 removed
I tbsp grated Cheddar cheese
I tsp chopped fresh cilantro
 (optional)

• In blender or food processor, pulse chicken, avocado, cheese and cilantro (if using) to achieve desired consistency.

Yield: 1 serving

ZUCCHINI CHICKEN AND CHEESE

I tbsp olive oil
1/4 onion, diced
I zucchini, washed, trimmed and
 diced
1/2 Poached Chicken Breast
 (recipe, page 48)
1/2 cup grated Cheddar cheese
 (2 oz)
1/3 cup chopped fresh parsley
 (optional)
3 tbsp high-fat (above 3%) plain
 yogurt
2 tomatoes, washed, skinned,
 seeded and diced (recipe,
 page 60)

• In frying pan, heat oil and sauté onion on medium heat until translucent, about 5 minutes. Add zucchini and continue to sauté until thoroughly cooked, 20 to 25 minutes. Remove from heat and cool.
• In blender or food processor, pulse zucchini mixture with chicken, cheese, parsley (if using), yogurt and tomatoes to achieve desired consistency.
• Fill ice cube trays and freeze.

Yield: 16 cubes

OKANAGAN SUMMER CHICKEN

The intriguing combination of creamy corn and peaches makes this dish a delectable treat.

2 peaches, washed

I cob corn, husked and kernels
    removed

1/2 Poached Chicken Breast
    (recipe, page 48)

• In saucepan, plunge peaches into boiling water for 30 seconds. Remove with slotted spoon and cool. Slit skin with a knife and remove. Cut peaches into quarters, removing pit.

• In steamer, steam peaches and corn over boiling water for 5 minutes. Reserve leftover cooking water.

• In blender or food processor, purée peaches, corn and chicken to achieve desired consistency. If purée seems too thick, add either leftover cooking water or unsweetened apple juice, 1 tbsp at a time.

• Fill ice cube trays and freeze.

Yield: 12 cubes

SUMMER SALAD

2 oz Poached Chicken Breast
    (1/8 of whole) (recipe, page 48)

I slice avocado, washed, skin
    removed

I slice mango, washed, skin
    removed

• In blender or food processor, pulse chicken, avocado and mango to desired consistency. Serve.

Yield: 1 serving

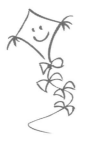

PASTA AND RICE

As your baby begins to declare her independence, pasta and sauce is a good choice. Although messy, individual pieces can be grasped by little hands. Newspaper under the high chair facilitates a quick cleanup.

Many of the vegetable purées make delicious pasta sauces. Heat 2 cubes of your baby's favorite vegetable purée and mix with 1 oz cooked pasta and 1 tbsp grated cheese.

TOMATO AND CHEESE PASTA

1/4 cup (2 oz) dried pasta
2 cubes Tomato Sauce (recipe, page 61)
1 tbsp grated mozzarella cheese

• Defrost cubes of tomato sauce.
• In saucepan, cook pasta in boiling water. Drain pasta and rinse under cool water.
• In separate saucepan, combine tomato sauce, pasta and mozzarella cheese over low heat. Stir until cheese melts.
• Using blender or food processor, pulse to desired consistency.

Yield: 1 serving

PASTA WITH FLORETS AND CHEESE

1/4 cup (2 oz) dried pasta
2 cubes Florets and Cheese Sauce (recipe, page 90)

• Defrost cubes of Florets and Cheese Sauce.
• In saucepan, cook pasta in boiling water; drain.
• In separate saucepan, combine pasta and sauce over low heat until pasta is thoroughly coated.
• In blender or food processor, pulse mixture to desired consistency.

Yield: 1 serving

BABY'S VEGETABLE RISOTTO

I cup arborio rice

1/2 onion, diced

2 tbsp olive oil

I baby zucchini, washed and
    trimmed

1/2 sweet red pepper, washed,
    peeled with potato peeler

I small carrot, washed, peeled and
    trimmed

2 1/2 cups Salt-Free Chicken
    Stock (recipe, page 66)

I cup grated Parmesan (4 oz)

• Rinse rice and set aside.

• In a large frying pan, sauté onion in oil over medium heat for 5 minutes. Meanwhile, dice both zucchini and pepper into small-bite-sized pieces; grate carrot. Add zucchini, pepper and carrot to frying pan and continue to sauté until vegetables are soft, 10 to 12 minutes.

• Add rice and 1/4 cup chicken stock; simmer over medium heat. As the rice becomes dry, add more chicken stock to keep the rice moist, and stir after each addition. Chicken stock should be added in small increments throughout the entire cooking process, 20 to 25 minutes. When rice is cooked it should be just tender.

• During the last 2 minutes of cooking time, add cheese; stir until cheese melts. (Do not be tempted to add extra chicken stock, as it will cause risotto to clump.)

• Cool risotto. Fill ice cube trays and freeze.

• *Tip:* For younger babies you may choose to use a blender or food processor to pulse risotto to desired consistency.

Yield: 16 cubes

FROM EIGHT MONTHS

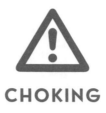

CHOKING

Each year many Canadian children die as a result of choking on food or small objects. That's why it is important to ensure all food is well puréed for babies, well mashed for older babies, or cut in small pieces for toddlers.

BABIES AND TODDLERS MUST ALWAYS BE SUPERVISED WHEN EATING.

Some foods are known to be associated with choking and should be carefully prepared, or avoided (see Proceed with Caution, page 57). Small toys, marbles, latex balloons and plastic bags can also cause choking. Parents and caregivers should be familiar with life-saving techniques and take a child safety course such as those offered by St. John Ambulance (see Appendix I).

ASSESSING THE CHOKING CHILD

1. If the child is breathing and able to make sounds or speak it is likely that natural coughing will dislodge the object. Additional maneuvers could be potentially dangerous.
2. If the child is not breathing, coughing or making sounds, back blows or chest thrusts are recommended (depending on the child's age).

TECHNIQUE IF THE CHOKING CHILD IS YOUNGER THAN 1 YEAR OF AGE:

1. Call an ambulance.
2. Place the infant facedown at an angle of 60 degrees along the rescuer's forearm and ensure head and neck are stabilized. For a larger infant, place facedown on the rescuer's lap with head firmly supported and held lower than the trunk.
3. Administer four back blows rapidly between the shoulder blades using the heel of the hand.
4. If no relief, turn the infant over and place on a firm surface. Deliver four rapid chest thrusts over the breastbone using two fingers.
5. If no relief, open the infant's mouth by grasping the tongue and jaw between the fingers and lifting up. By removing the tongue from the back of the throat it may be possible to visualize the object and remove with a finger. If no object is seen, blindly trying to remove the obstruction with a finger may lodge it further and should be avoided.
6. If there is no breathing, give two breaths by mouth-to-mouth or mouth-to-nose resuscitation and continue these maneuvers while calling for an ambulance.

TECHNIQUE IF THE VICTIM IS A SMALL CHILD OLDER THAN 1 YEAR:

1. Call an ambulance.
2. Administer the Heimlich maneuver. This requires the child to be placed on his back on a table or the floor. Place the heel of one hand in the midline between the belly button and rib cage. Next place the other hand over the first and deliver 6 to 10 inward and upward thrusts. This should be done gently in small children.
3. If no relief, open the mouth by grasping the tongue and the lower jaw between the fingers and lifting up. If you can see the object, attempt to dislodge it; do not attempt blindly.
4. If the child is not breathing, give two breaths by mouth-to-mouth resuscitation and repeat the maneuvers above.

BROCCOLI RISOTTO

I cup arborio rice

2 cups broccoli florets, washed

2 1/2 cups Salt-Free Chicken
   Stock (recipe, page 66)

1/2 onion, diced

I tbsp olive oil

I cup grated Parmesan cheese
   (4 oz)

I tbsp salt-free butter

• Rinse rice and set aside.

• In saucepan, blanch broccoli in boiling chicken stock for 4 to 5 minutes; drain and set stock aside. (This preserves nutrients that would otherwise be lost.) Once cool, chop broccoli into baby-bite-size pieces.

• Meanwhile, in frying pan, heat oil and sauté onion over medium heat until translucent, about 5 minutes. Add rice and 1/4 cup chicken stock and cook. As the rice becomes dry, add chicken stock, keeping the rice moist; stir after each addition. Chicken stock should be added in small increments throughout the entire cooking process, 20 to 25 minutes.

• During the last 5 minutes of cooking time, add broccoli and stir gently.

• When rice is cooked it should be just tender. (Do not be tempted to add extra chicken stock, as it will cause the rice to clump.) Once cooked, remove from heat and stir in cheese and butter. Allow to cool.

• Fill ice cube trays and freeze.

• *Tip:* For younger babies you may choose to pulse risotto in food processor to achieve desired consistency.

Yield: 16 cubes

PESTICIDES AND HORMONES IN PRODUCE AND MEAT

Controversy regarding hormone and pesticide use has caused many people to go "organic." Is this extra expense necessary? As of 1998, Canada has banned the use of growth hormones in cattle. (The American Food and Drug Administration and other regulatory agencies have concluded that the growth hormone known as bovine somatotropin (bST) is a protein hormone and is inactivated when consumed by mouth. Furthermore the hormone is structurally unlike human growth hormone and therefore unable to affect human growth and development. Pesticides in produce are strictly researched and monitored by regulatory bodies. Only those pesticides not known to cause adverse effects at reasonable levels of consumption are approved.

Parents should not restrict produce consumption because of pesticide fears as there is overwhelming scientific consensus that the health benefits of eating produce far outweigh any possible pesticide risks. To minimize risk, choose produce free of dirt, cuts, insect holes or mold, wash produce thoroughly in water and remove outer skin or leaves, and eat a variety of foods. There is no evidence that "organically grown" foods are safer or more nutritious than foods conventionally grown. In fact, many organic growers use "environmental" pesticides such as sulphur, nicotine and copper, and the relative risks of these pesticides compared with synthetic ones is unknown.

LASAGNA MASH

I can (14 oz) diced tomatoes

1/4 cup water

8 cubes stewing beef

1/4 onion, diced

I carrot, washed, peeled and
   sliced

1/2 cup (4 oz) macaroni or other
   dried pasta

I tbsp chopped fresh basil
   (optional)

1/3 cup grated mozzarella cheese
   (1.5 oz)

1/2 cup cottage cheese

• In saucepan, combine tomatoes, water, beef, onion, carrot and pasta; bring to a boil. Reduce heat and simmer, partially covered, stirring occasionally, until meat is thoroughly cooked, 25 to 30 minutes. The consistency should be that of a thick stew. If you feel there is too much liquid, remove the lid for the last 5 to 10 minutes of cooking.
• Remove from heat; add basil (if using) and cheeses. Stir until cheese melts.

• In blender or food processor, pulse mixture to desired consistency.
• Fill ice cube trays and freeze.

Yield: 16 to 18 cubes

QUICK AND EASY PASTA AND CHEESE

This simple recipe is a healthy alternative to store-bought macaroni and cheese.

1/4 cup (2 oz) cooked pasta

1/3 cup grated Cheddar cheese
   (1.5 oz)

I tbsp breast milk or formula
   (3.25% milk after age 12
   months)

• In saucepan over low heat, stir together pasta, cheese and milk. Mix until cheese melts and pasta is thoroughly coated.
• In blender or food processor, pulse the mixture to desired consistency.

Yield: 1 serving

TINY TOT'S TUNA PASTA

The sauce for this recipe can be either pre-mixed with pasta, or frozen separately and mixed before serving.

1/4 onion, diced

1 tbsp olive oil

1 tbsp tomato paste

1 can (14 oz) diced tomatoes

1 tin white tuna (water-packed), drained

1 tbsp chopped fresh parsley (optional)

1 1/2 cups (12 oz) dried pasta, cooked

• In frying pan, heat oil; sauté onion until translucent, about 5 minutes. Add tomato paste and tomatoes. Mix well; cover with lid and simmer for 5 minutes.

• Add tuna and stir; continue to simmer, stirring occasionally, for another 20 minutes.

• Add parsley (if using); stir.

• In blender or food processor, purée pasta and tomato mixture to desired consistency.

• Fill ice cube trays and freeze.

Yield: 16 to 18 cubes

PAVAROTTI AND PASTA

Ambience may be as important as the food itself when it comes to a toddler's appetite. Make an effort to eat together as a family, and try to maintain a pleasant atmosphere throughout mealtime. This takes the focus off the toddler and reduces his temptation to refuse the meal. Peaceful dinner music may also help the toddler to see mealtime as a relaxing, positive experience.

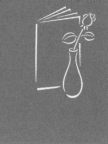

CHICKEN AND VEGETABLE RISOTTO

I cup arborio rice

2 tbsp olive oil

1/2 chicken breast, minced in food
    processor (or 1/2 lb ground
    chicken)

1/2 onion, diced

I small carrot, washed, peeled
    and grated

2 stalks celery, washed, trimmed
    and diced

2 1/2 cups Salt-Free Chicken
    Stock (recipe, page 66)

I cup grated Parmesan cheese
    (4 oz)

I tbsp chopped fresh parsley
    (optional)

• Rinse rice and set aside.

• In frying pan, sauté chicken over medium heat in 1 tbsp of oil until there are no traces of pink, 5 to 6 minutes. Set chicken aside.

• Using the same pan, sauté onion, carrot and celery in remaining tbsp of oil until onion is translucent, about 5 minutes.

• Add rice and 1/4 cup chicken stock; cook over medium heat.

As rice becomes dry, slowly add chicken stock, keeping the rice moist and stirring after each addition. After 10 minutes the chicken should be mixed into the rice. Chicken stock should be added in small increments throughout the entire cooking process, 20 to 25 minutes. When rice is cooked it should be just tender.

• During the last 2 minutes of cooking time, add cheese and parsley (if using). Stir until cheese melts. (Do not be tempted to add extra chicken stock, as it will cause risotto to clump.) Remove from heat.

• Add parsley (if using); stir. Allow to cool.

• Fill ice cube trays and freeze.

• *Tip:* For younger babies you may choose to use a blender or food processor to purée risotto to desired consistency before freezing.

Yield: 16 to 18 cubes

FISH

Fish is easy to cook, high in protein and one of the few sources of omega-3 fatty acids. Fish is also easy for your baby to chew, whether served on its own or puréed with vegetables.

Baking in foil is the simplest way to cook fish—allowing it to cook in its own juices. The easiest way to remove the skin is to cook the fish with the skin intact and then gently remove it when done. When done, fish will be firm to touch, opaque throughout and flake easily with a fork.

When serving fish to a baby you must check carefully for bones. The only way to be sure there are no bones is to flake the cooked fish apart with your fingers. You can never be too careful about bones when serving fish to your baby.

FISH OIL AND ASTHMA

In addition to having a low incidence of heart disease, populations that regularly consume oily, marine fish also have low incidences of certain inflammatory diseases. Early clinical trials have shown fish oil to be beneficial in diseases such as rheumatoid arthritis, psoriasis, cystic fibrosis and inflammatory bowel disease. The beneficial properties of oily fish are thought to be due to an omega-3 fatty acid known as EPA (eicosapentaenoic acid), which works as a potent anti-inflammatory. This theory has provoked several studies into the benefit of fish oil for asthma, a chronic inflammatory disease of the airway. The most promising result was a study conducted in Australia, showing an almost one-third reduction in the incidence of asthma among children who consumed fresh oily fish more than once a week.

FROM EIGHT MONTHS

WHAT ARE OMEGA-3 FATTY ACIDS?

Omega-3 fatty acids are highly unsaturated long-chain fatty acids thought to significantly reduce the development of heart disease in adults and to improve cognitive function and vision in infants. It has long been known that Greenland Inuit, Japanese and Scandinavian populations have much lower rates of heart disease. The common feature among these populations is the consumption of fish, in particular cold-water marine fish, such as salmon, trout, tuna and sardines. The substance in oily fish has now been identified as omega-3 fatty acid. Further research has revealed that 40 percent of the polyunsaturated fatty acids that make up the brain and 60 percent of those that make up the retina are a type of omega-3 known as DHA (docosahexaenoic acid).

At one time, humans consumed far higher quantities of omega-3 fatty acids than we do today. This is because prior to the agricultural revolution, humans consumed wild animals that grazed on omega-3 rich plants. Interestingly, human milk contains omega-3 fatty acids at a ratio to other fats similar to that in our ancestors' diet. Today, animals raised for consumption are fed diets such as corn and soybean, which are very low in omega-3. Consequently the ratio of omega-3 to other fats in our diet has been reduced 10 to 30 fold. Omega-3 is present in significant quantities in oily fish, human breast milk, flax seed, omega-3 eggs and, to a lesser extent, in regular eggs. Consequently, for those who do not consume fish, omega-3 levels are far below recommended intakes. To increase intake and reap the benefits of omega-3, adults should consume 2 to 3 servings of fish per week.

WEST COAST SALMON

8 oz salmon fillet

I tbsp chopped fresh dill (optional)

I tbsp finely diced onion

dash lemon juice

I potato, washed, peeled and cut
 in cubes

I tbsp breast milk or formula
 (approx) (3.25% milk after age
 I2 months)

• Place fish on tinfoil. Coat with dill (if using), onion and dash of lemon juice. Wrap in foil and bake in 375°F oven until thoroughly cooked, about 20 minutes.

• Open foil and allow to cool. Flake fish apart with fingers to remove skin and bones. Set fish aside; save cooking juices.

• In pot of boiling water, cook potato until tender, about 20 minutes. In blender or food processor, purée potato, fish, cooking juices and milk. If mixture seems too thick, add extra milk to achieve desired consistency.

• Fill ice cube trays and freeze.

Yield: 12 cubes

SOLE WITH SALSA AND CHEESE

8 oz sole fillet

2 tomatoes, skinned and seeded
 and diced (recipe, page 60)

I tbsp finely diced onion

I tbsp chopped fresh parsley
 (optional)

I/2 cup grated Cheddar cheese
 (2 oz)

• Place fish on tinfoil.

• In bowl, mix tomatoes, onion and parsley (if using). Coat fish with this tomato salsa and wrap in foil. Bake in 375°F oven until fish is thoroughly cooked, about 20 minutes.

• Open foil to allow cooling. Flake fish apart with fingers to remove skin and bones.

• In blender or food processor, pulse fish, tomato salsa and cheese to achieve desired consistency.

• Fill ice cube trays and freeze.

Yield: 10 to 12 cubes

SOLE, VEGETABLES AND CHEESE

This is a fabulous way to introduce your baby to fish.

10 oz sole fillet or any white fish
Dash lemon juice
I tbsp finely diced onion
2 cups broccoli florets, washed
2 carrots, washed, peeled and
    sliced
I tsp of flour (approx)
I tsp butter (approx)
1/2 cup breast milk or formula
    (3.25% milk after age I2 months)
1/2 cup grated Cheddar cheese
    (2 oz)

• Place fish on tinfoil. Sprinkle with lemon juice and onion. Wrap fish in foil. Bake in 375°F oven until fish is thoroughly cooked, about 20 minutes.
• Open foil to allow cooling. Flake fish apart with fingers to remove both skin and bones. Set fish aside; reserve cooking juices.
• Meanwhile, in steamer, cook vegetables over boiling water until tender; set aside.
• In saucepan, whisk flour and butter together over medium heat until paste forms. Add 1/4 cup milk, whisking constantly until lumps disappear. Add cheese and remainder of milk, whisking until cheese melts.
• Add cooking juices to pan; whisk until sauce thickens.
• In blender or food processor, purée vegetables, sauce and fish to desired consistency.
• Fill ice cube trays and freeze.

Yield: 14 cubes

OMEGA-3 AND BEHAVIOR AND LEARNING

Preliminary studies have shown a correlation between the symptoms that characterize attention deficit hyperactivity disorder (ADHD) and blood levels of omega-3 fatty acids. Boys with lower levels of omega-3 fatty acids showed more problems with behavior and learning than those with higher levels of omega-3 fatty acids.

RED SNAPPER SALSA PROVENÇAL

12 oz red snapper fillet, bones
    removed
1/4 red onion, finely diced
2 tomatoes, skinned, seeded and
    diced (recipe, page 60)
1 tbsp chopped fresh parsley
    (optional)
1 tbsp chopped fresh basil
    (optional)
1 potato, baked, skin removed

• Place fish on tinfoil. In bowl mix onion, tomatoes and herbs (if using). Coat fish with this tomato salsa. Wrap fish in foil.
• Bake in 375°F oven until fish is thoroughly cooked, about 25 minutes. Open foil to allow cooling. Flake fish apart with fingers to remove skin and bones.
• In blender or food processor, purée fish, salsa and potato to achieve desired consistency.
• Fill ice cube trays and freeze.

Yield: 14 cubes

TUNA SALAD

1/4 tin white tuna (water-packed),
    drained
1 tbsp cucumber, washed, peeled
    and finely diced
1/4 avocado, washed, skin
    removed, pitted and mashed
1 tsp chopped fresh cilantro
    (optional)

• In bowl, combine ingredients and serve.
• *Tip:* For younger babies you may choose to use a blender or food processor to purée to achieve desired consistency.

Yield: 1 serving

SALMON AND VEGETABLES WITH CREAMY DILL SAUCE

10 oz salmon fillet, bones and skin
   removed
1 tbsp lemon juice
1 tbsp diced onion (approx)
2 carrots, washed, peeled and
   chopped
2 cups broccoli florets, washed
1 rounded tsp butter
1 rounded tsp flour
1/3 cup breast milk or formula
   (3.25% milk after age 12
   months)
1 tbsp chopped fresh dill

• Place salmon on tinfoil. Sprinkle with lemon and onion.
• Wrap in foil and bake in 375°F oven until salmon is thoroughly cooked, about 20 minutes. Open foil to cool. Flake fish apart with fingers to remove both skin and bones. Set fish aside; save juices.
• In steamer, cook vegetables over boiling water until tender.
• Meanwhile, in saucepan, whisk butter and flour together over medium heat until paste forms. Add milk, whisking constantly until lumps disappear. Then add dill and cooking juices, continuing to simmer until sauce thickens.
• In blender or food processor, pulse vegetables, salmon and sauce to desired consistency.

Yield: 14 to 16 cubes

SMART SARDINES

Sardines are one of the richest sources of omega-3 fatty acids. The ingredients in this recipe can be easily mashed for older babies.

1 can (125 oz) sardines packed in
   tomato sauce
2 cups broccoli florets, washed
1 large potato, baked, skin
   removed

• In steamer, cook broccoli over boiling water until tender.
• In blender or food processor, pulse sardines, potato and broccoli to achieve desired consistency.
• Fill ice cube trays and freeze.

Yield 14 to 16 cubes

BREAKFAST IDEAS

Commercial baby cereals are the best choice for baby's breakfast, and should form the staple of the diet in the first year because they are heavily fortified with iron. It is advisable to serve commercial baby cereal well into the second year of life and until baby has a reliable intake of iron from other sources. At 8 to 10 months of age, baby can be introduced to alternative breakfast cereals for occasional variety; however, they should not replace baby cereal. Look for toddler cereals that are iron-fortified and help to promote self-feeding skills. The vast majority of adult cereals, including the ones whose names "sound" healthy, have excessive sugar, salt and unwanted trans fats.

BANANA CRUNCH

Cornflakes contain traces of soybeans and therefore should not be consumed by babies suspected of having a soy allergy. If you have a family history of allergies, delay introducing soy products until baby is 1 year old.

1/3 cup cornflakes

1/3 banana, mashed

I tbsp high-fat (over 3%) plain
    yogurt

1/4 cup breast milk or formula
    (3.25% milk after age 12
    months)

• In bowl, mash cornflakes and banana together with a fork. Add yogurt and enough milk to achieve desired consistency.

Yield: 1 serving

YOGURT APPLE CEREAL

You can make this with any of the fruit purées, or with mashed banana.

1/4 cup Cheerios
2 cubes Apple Purée (recipe, page 30)
1/3 cup high-fat (over 3%) plain yogurt

• In bowl, crush Cheerios with a fork.
• Defrost 2 cubes apple purée. Mix with Cheerios and yogurt. Serve.

Yield: 1 serving

DRIED FRUIT CEREAL

I cube mixed Dried Fruit Purée (recipe, page 57)
1/4 cup Cheerios
1/3 cup high-fat (over 3%) plain yogurt

• In bowl, crush Cheerios with a fork.
• Defrost 1 cube fruit purée. Mix with Cheerios and yogurt. Serve.

Yield: 1 serving

BALANCING FIBER

Increasing fiber is a main principle in reducing fat intake and preventing both heart and bowel disease in adults. In babies less than 2 years of age, however, promoting an excessively high-fiber diet may be detrimental. Babies depend on a large intake of fats as the primary source of energy for rapid growth and brain development. Since fiber acts as a bulking agent, excessively high intakes may result in decreased intake of other food groups, most importantly fats. A healthy approach to fiber intake for your baby is several servings per week of a variety of fruits, whole grains and legumes. After 2 years of age fiber intake should be increased.

BANANA PORRIDGE

1/4 cup instant porridge oats
1/2 cup breast milk or formula
    (3.25% milk after age 12
    months)
1/3 banana, mashed

• In saucepan, combine milk and oats over medium heat; simmer for 5 minutes, stirring occasionally.
• Mix with mashed banana. If consistency is too thick, add extra milk as needed. Serve.

Yield: 1 serving

APPLE PORRIDGE

1/4 cup instant porridge oats
1/2 cup breast milk or formula
    (3.25% milk at age 12 months)
1/2 apple, washed, peeled and
    grated
1 tbsp raisins

• In saucepan, combine oats, milk, apple and raisins over medium heat; simmer for 5 minutes, stirring occasionally. If consistency is too thick, add extra milk as needed. Serve.

Yield: 1 serving

SHREDDED WHEAT AND APPLES

You can experiment with this recipe by substituting either mashed banana or any of the fruit purées for the apple. Shredded Wheat should not be consumed by babies who have been diagnosed with wheat allergy or gluten intolerance.

1 brick Shredded Wheat
1/2 sweet apple, washed, peeled
    and grated
1/2 cup breast milk or formula
    (3.25% milk after age 12
    months)

• Thoroughly crumble Shredded Wheat. Mix with grated apple. Add milk and stir to achieve desired consistency. Serve.

Yield: 1 serving

MANAGING GASTROENTERITIS

At some point your child may experience diarrhea and vomiting and be diagnosed with gastroenteritis, as most children under age 3 have at least one episode per year. Gastroenteritis refers to an infection of the gastrointestinal tract, which results in diarrhea, vomiting, decreased appetite and possibly fever. By far the most common cause of gastroenteritis is viral, resulting in mild symptoms of diarrhea and vomiting without serious dehydration or illness. The exception is Rotavirus, which may cause more severe symptoms with fever and marked dehydration. Other causes of gastroenteritis are bacterial, often acquired from infected food or water, or giardia. Bacterial infections may result in blood in the stool and more serious symptoms.

In general, viral and mild bacterial infections may last 5 to 10 days. During the illness it is important to keep your child well hydrated, something you can monitor by checking for wet diapers. Recommendations from the Canadian Paediatric Society and The American Academy of Pediatrics have re-evaluated earlier positions on milk intake. Experts now believe that milk should be continued throughout the illness and does not affect the severity or duration of diarrhea in mild to moderate cases. In rare cases temporary lactose intolerance (lasting anywhere from 3 to 10 days) may develop and diarrhea will become much worse. If this occurs, your doctor may recommend an alternative to cow's-milk-based formula.

The question surrounding what to eat during the illness has been under considerable debate. In the past, doctors recommended limited diets. Today, however, the thinking is that a wide diet of breads, rice, potatoes, meat, yogurt, fruits and vegetables are better tolerated than fatty foods or foods high in sugar content such as fruit juice or soft drinks.

The most effective means of preventing spread to other family members is frequent hand washing by everyone. Consult your doctor for further advice regarding gastroenteritis or for serious symptoms such as blood in the stool, fever or persistence of symptoms. Babies under 1 year of age should be evaluated by a doctor if symptoms persist longer than 24 hours.

FINGER FOOD

From 8 months of age your baby may express an interest in feeding herself: this is the time to introduce finger foods. When introducing such foods for the first time choose soft fruits (bananas, peaches or pears) or steamed vegetables. Teething babies may enjoy eating Melba toast, dry bread crusts, bagels or frozen bananas. Starting a meal with finger foods is often a good way to distract baby while the main course is being prepared.

Your baby should eat finger foods only when sitting upright and supervised by an adult. Some foods are considered risky because they can cause choking and therefore should be avoided by both babies and toddlers. See Proceed with Caution (page 57). Remember when serving fruit to peel and remove both the seeds and the pit.

At around 1 year of age it is not unusual for your baby to refuse to be fed by you altogether. Often the best way to encourage your baby to eat is to offer a variety of finger foods. At this stage your baby may enjoy eating pieces of cooked meat or cubes of cheese. A well-balanced meal can be made entirely of finger foods. An easy way to prepare such meals in advance is to poach one chicken breast, and steam half a head of broccoli and two carrots. Cut up chicken, broccoli and carrots into finger-size pieces, divide into individual portions and freeze in freezer bags. *To serve:* Defrost. Heat in oven until warm.

What follows are some ideas for a smorgasbord of finger foods.

FRUIT Peeled raw fruit such as bananas, pears, peaches, papaya or blueberries are good introductory finger foods. Seedless grapes should be cut lengthways several times. Harder fruits such as apples can be grated or served in larger pieces that your baby can hold and chew on. (Cold apples or frozen bananas can help soothe sore gums.)

125

Dried fruit is rich in iron and many toddlers find it fun to chew. Remember to always brush your baby's teeth after serving dried fruit.

VEGETABLES Steamed cauliflower, broccoli, beans or peas are tasty. Carrots should be served either soft-cooked or grated. Cherry tomatoes cut in quarters, shredded lettuce, ripe avocados and celery with the strands removed can all be served raw. Potatoes cut in wedges and roasted are a healthy alternative to french fries.

BREADS AND CEREALS You may introduce toast, whole-grain crackers and rice cakes at this stage. Cooked pasta can be served either on its own or with a thick sauce. Whole-grain cereal such as Cheerios, cornflakes or Spoon-Size Shredded Wheat can be served without milk. If your baby begins to lose interest in your purées, try serving them as a dip with either toast strips or precooked vegetable sticks.

MEATS AND PROTEINS By 1 year of age your baby may enjoy eating small pieces of cooked chicken, beef or fish. Whatever meat you are cooking for dinner, make sure there will be some left over for baby's lunch the next day. The fish sticks and chicken fingers in this book are popular. Serve them with homemade Tomato Sauce (recipe, page 61) or some of the vegetable purées. Dipping fish sticks into Florets and Cheese Sauce (recipe, page 90) is an entertaining way for your baby to eat a well-balanced meal.

DAIRY PRODUCTS Cheese can be served either grated or cut in cubes, and most babies enjoy cheese melted on bread cut into strips.

WEEK 1

DAY 1

Breakfast	Breast or Bottle, Shredded Wheat and Apples
Mid-A.M. Snack	Banana and Whole-Wheat Toast Strips
Lunch	Breast or Bottle, Sole, Vegetables and Cheese
Mid-P.M. Snack	Breast or Bottle
Dinner	Tuscan Tomato and Chick-peas
Before Bed	Breast or Bottle

DAY 2

Breakfast	Breast or Bottle, Mixed-Grain Baby Cereal
Mid-A.M. Snack	Papaya and Cottage Cheese
Lunch	Breast or Bottle, Minestrone, Whole-Wheat Toast Strips
Mid-P.M. Snack	Breast or Bottle
Dinner	Baja Chicken Salad, Melon
Before Bed	Breast or Bottle

DAY 3

Breakfast	Breast or Bottle, Banana Porridge
Mid-A.M. Snack	Tropical Smoothie
Lunch	Breast or Bottle, Pork and Apple Purée
Mid-P.M. Snack	Breast or Bottle
Dinner	Roasted Veggie Mash Purée, Papaya
Before Bed	Breast or Bottle

DAY 4

Breakfast	Breast or Bottle, Mixed-Grain Cereal (Rice) and Mashed Pear
Mid-A.M. Snack	Peeled Apple Slices
Lunch	Breast or Bottle, Spinach and Cheese Purée, Yogurt
Mid-P.M. Snack	Breast or Bottle
Dinner	Sole with Salsa & Cheese, Mashed Banana
Before Bed	Breast or Bottle

DAY 5

Breakfast	Breast or Bottle, Single-Grain Cereal (Rice) and Mashed Papaya
Mid-A.M. Snack	Whole-Wheat Toast Strips and Cheese Slices
Lunch	Lasagna Mash, Banana
Mid-P.M. Snack	Breast or Bottle
Dinner	Vichyssoise, Melon
Before Bed	Breast or Bottle

SAMPLE WEEKLY MEAL PLANNER: FROM EIGHT TO TWELVE MONTHS

WEEK I continued

DAY 6

Breakfast	Breast or Bottle, Apple Cinnamon Porridge
Mid-A.M. Snack	Yogurt
Lunch	Shepherd's Mash
Mid-P.M. Snack	Breast or Bottle
Dinner	Baked Tomato and Zucchini au Gratin, Apple Slices
Before Bed	Breast or Bottle

DAY 7

Breakfast	Breast or Bottle, Single-Grain Baby Cereal (Rice) and Apple
Mid-A.M. Snack	Fruit Smoothie
Lunch	Breast or Bottle, Broccoli Risotto, Pear Slices
Mid-P.M. Snack	Breast or Bottle
Dinner	Brown Rice and Vegetables, Melon
Before Bed	Breast or Bottle

SAMPLE WEEKLY MEAL PLANNER: FROM EIGHT TO TWELVE MONTHS

WEEK 2

DAY I

Breakfast	Breast or Bottle, Single-Grain Baby Cereal (Rice)
Mid-A.M. Snack	Whole-Wheat Toast Strips Dipped in Florets and Cheese Sauce
Lunch	Breast or Bottle, Navy Beans, Yogurt
Mid-P.M. Snack	Breast or Bottle
Dinner	Maxwell's Minted Lamb and Steamed Vegetable Sticks
Before Bed	Breast or Bottle

DAY 2

Breakfast	Breast or Bottle, Mixed-Grain Baby Cereal and Mashed Pear
Mid-A.M. Snack	Melon
Lunch	Breast or Bottle, Chicken Noodle Stew, Yogurt
Mid-P.M. Snack	Breast or Bottle
Dinner	Barley Risotto, Banana
Before Bed	Breast or Bottle

SAMPLE WEEKLY MEAL PLANNER: FROM EIGHT TO TWELVE MONTHS

WEEK 2 continued

DAY 3

Breakfast	Breast or Bottle, Banana Crunch
Mid-A.M. Snack	Steamed Vegetable Sticks
Lunch	Breast or Bottle, Shepherd's Mash, Blueberries
Mid-P.M. Snack	Breast or Bottle
Dinner	Tuna Salad, Banana
Before Bed	Breast or Bottle

DAY 4

Breakfast	Breast or Bottle, Mixed-Grain Baby Cereal
Mid-A.M. Snack	Down Under Fruit Salad
Lunch	Breast or Bottle, Red Snapper Salsa Provençal
Mid-P.M. Snack	Breast or Bottle
Dinner	Spinach and Cheese, Liz's Couscous
Before Bed	Breast or Bottle

DAY 5

Breakfast	Breast or Bottle, Banana Porridge
Mid-A.M. Snack	Fruit Smoothie
Lunch	Breast or Bottle, Thanksgiving Dinner
Mid-P.M. Snack	Breast or Bottle
Dinner	Minestrone, Papaya
Before Bed	Breast or Bottle

DAY 6

Breakfast	Breast or Bottle, Single-Grain Baby Cereal (Wheat) and Mashed Pear
Mid-A.M. Snack	Whole-Wheat Cheerios
Lunch	Breast or Bottle, Green Lentils, Whole-Wheat Toast Strips
Mid-P.M. Snack	Breast or Bottle
Dinner	Baby Chicken, Yogurt
Before Bed	Breast or Bottle

DAY 7

Breakfast	Breast or Bottle, Yogurt Cereal
Mid-A.M. Snack	Vegetable Sticks
Lunch	Breast or Bottle, Summer Chicken, Banana
Mid-P.M. Snack	Breast or Bottle
Dinner	West Coast Salmon
Before Bed	Breast or Bottle

Toddlers

In your child's second year of life, you will find it important to adapt to her individual appetite. Meeting these requirements may mean frequent feedings throughout the day; your child may require 4 to 6 feedings in addition to milk intake. At this stage the goal is to provide nutritious food from a variety of food groups.

The statement of the Joint Working Group of the Canadian Paediatric Society, Dietitians of Canada, and Health Canada recommends small, frequent, energy-dense feedings. For now, put aside the idea of three square meals a day and respect your toddler's hunger and willingness to eat. Appetite varies according to growth, activity, fatigue, frustration, illness and social setting. Toddlers should be given the opportunity to ask for more if they are hungry and to say "enough" when they are not.

At this stage many parents find success with meals made up of finger foods, while others find their toddlers are still enjoying mushy purées. It is not uncommon for toddlers to advance from preferring mashed carrots one week to soft-cooked carrot sticks the next. If your child refuses a meal, try not to get frustrated. Take the meal away and offer a snack later. Avoid the temptation to focus on the intake of a single meal. Instead, evaluate your toddler's nutritional intake over several days to weeks. It is important to be flexible and sensitive to changing preferences. Patience and a sense of humor are vital; this can be a frustrating time for all.

When out and about, your toddler does not have to subsist on a diet of convenience food. With a little preparation he can enjoy healthy snacks and meals all day long. Whole-wheat toast strips, whole-grain crackers, cereal, rice crackers, steamed vegetable sticks, fruit and chunks of cheese can be easily packed in airtight containers. Bring a cup and bottle of water or juice. On a hot day, freeze the bottle before leaving; this will help to keep the food cool, and the drink will melt as the day progresses.

Creative (and sometimes silly!) presentation is effective. Drawing a funny face on a bowl of porridge can be a hit with fussy eaters, or, instead of sprinkling berries on a bowl of cereal, arrange them into a happy face. Food decorating can add pizzazz to any meal. For example, slices of hard-boiled eggs, cherry tomatoes and olives make wonderful eyes. Steamed broccoli florets or bean sprouts become a wild head of hair. A steamed carrot stick becomes the nose, and slices of apple or orange form the mouth. Toddlers delight in eating these funny faces. Be imaginative!

The following recipes are designed to be made in bulk and frozen in airtight containers. This method facilitates the serving of convenient, individual toddler meals. For many of the following recipes you will need 5 small, freezer-safe, airtight containers, or you can use muffin tins covered with plastic wrap.

VEGETABLE RAGOUT

Vegetable Ragout is an appealing meal for toddlers who like spaghetti but refuse to eat their vegetables. This pasta sauce is designed to be made in bulk and frozen in either small airtight containers or ice cube trays, depending on which is more convenient for your child.

1/2 onion, cut in half

2 carrots, washed, trimmed and
   sliced

2 stalks celery, washed, trimmed
   and sliced

8 broccoli florets, washed

2 cloves garlic (whole)

I tbsp dried oregano

2 tbsp olive oil

I 1/2 lb ground beef

I can (5.5 oz) tomato paste

3 cans (each 14 oz) diced tomatoes

I bay leaf (optional)

1/2 cup chopped fresh basil
   (optional)

Parmesan cheese

• Using a blender or food processor, finely chop onion, carrots, celery, broccoli, garlic and oregano.

• Pour mixture into frying pan and sauté in oil for 10 minutes over medium heat.

• Crumble in ground beef and cook until no longer pink. Add tomato paste, stirring until mixture is thoroughly coated.

• Add tomatoes and bay leaf (if using); stir. Bring to a rapid boil, reduce heat and simmer for 45 minutes, stirring occasionally. During the last 10 minutes of cooking time, add basil (if using) and stir.

• Allow to cool. Pour into airtight containers or ice cube trays and freeze.

• *To serve:* Defrost in refrigerator, heat, pour over cooked pasta and sprinkle with Parmesan cheese to taste.

Yield: 5 to 6 small airtight containers

YUMMY CHICKEN FINGERS

Homemade chicken fingers are a tasty and healthy alternative to store-bought, which often contain additives and preservatives. Serve with homemade Tomato Sauce (recipe, page 61) or one of your baby's favorite vegetable purées. These fingers work equally well with or without cheese; however, cheese does add flavor.

1/2 chicken breast

2 cups crushed cornflakes

1/2 cup grated Parmesan cheese
   (optional) (2 oz)

2 eggs, beaten

1 tbsp olive oil

• Cut chicken breast across the width into 8 fingers.
• In plastic bag combine cornflakes and cheese. Using rolling pin, crush until cornflakes are the consistency of bread crumbs.
• In bowl, dip chicken fingers into beaten egg. Place fingers in bag, one at a time, and shake until thoroughly coated with cornflakes mixture.
• Spread oil on baking sheet and bake chicken fingers in 350°F oven for 10 minutes. Flip chicken and bake for another 10 to 12 minutes. When cooked, chicken fingers should be crispy and golden brown.
• *Bulk:* This recipe can be made in bulk and frozen in either airtight containers or freezer bags. To make in bulk, double the recipe and freeze before baking.
• *To serve:* Defrost in refrigerator. Cook as above.

Yield: 8 chicken fingers

BABY BEEFCAKES

1 lb ground beef

1 egg

1 medium potato, baked

1 small carrot, washed, peeled and
 grated finely

1 tbsp chopped fresh parsley
 (optional)

1 tbsp tomato paste

2 tbsp onion, diced finely

1 tbsp olive oil

• In large bowl, mix all ingredients except olive oil thoroughly. Shape into small patties. Spread oil on baking sheet. Place patties on sheet and flatten with fork.

• Bake in 350°F oven for 10 minutes on each side.

• Allow to cool; freeze in freezer bags.

• *To serve:* Defrost in refrigerator. Heat in 350°F oven until warm.

Yield: 18 patties

HALIBUT FISH STICKS

Halibut fish sticks are a healthy alternative to commercial fish sticks and can be made with any white fish. These fish sticks work equally well with or without cheese; however, cheese does add a tasty zest to the topping.

8 oz halibut, bones and skin
 removed

1/2 cup grated Parmesan cheese
 (2 oz)

2 cups cornflakes

2 eggs, beaten

1 tbsp olive oil

• Remove skin from fish. Cut into 8 sticks, remembering to look carefully for bones.

• Pour cornflakes and cheese into a plastic bag. Using a rolling pin, crush cornflakes until they are the consistency of bread crumbs.

• In small bowl, dip fish sticks into beaten eggs. Place in plastic bag, one by one, and shake until they are thoroughly coated with cornflakes.

• Spread oil on baking sheet

and bake fish sticks in 350°F oven for 10 minutes. Flip fish and bake for another 10 minutes. When ready, fish sticks should be crispy and golden brown.

• *Bulk:* This recipe can be made in bulk and frozen in either airtight containers or freezer bags. Double recipe and freeze prior to cooking.

• *To serve:* Defrost in refrigerator. Cook as above.

Yield: 8 fish sticks

GOURMET TUNA MELTS

The following recipe makes a wholesome lunch for the whole family. If only serving baby, just make 1 tuna melt.

1 tin white tuna (water-packed), drained

1 tbsp lemon juice

1 tbsp red onion, finely diced

1 tbsp chopped fresh dill

2 tbsp mayonnaise

4 slices whole-wheat bread

4 oz Cheddar cheese, thinly sliced

• In bowl, thoroughly combine tuna, lemon juice, onion, dill and mayonnaise.

• Turn oven temperature to broil. Lightly toast bread in oven (to prevent bread from going soggy when it is broiled with tuna).

• Spread toast with tuna and cheese. On baking sheet, broil in 400°F oven about 2 minutes or until cheese begins to bubble. Remove from oven and allow to cool.

• Remove crusts and cut in bite-size pieces to serve.

Yield: 4 tuna melts

CHOOSING SAFE FISH

Concerns about toxins from fish arose in the 1960s following serious fish-related mercury poisonings in Japan. No such incidents have occurred in North America; however, concerns about the level of mercury in fish are valid. The earth's crust and waste discharge from industry are the main sources of mercury absorbed by fish. Once consumed by humans, mercury can accumulate in the body. If mercury reaches toxic levels, the result can be damage to the nervous system. Nearly all fish contain mercury levels well below the safety limit of 1 part per million. Only a few exceed the limit; these species include shark, swordfish and very large tuna that are sold as steaks or sushi (not small tuna used for canning). Current U.S. Federal Guidelines and Ontario Ministry of the Environment advice for pregnant women and children under 15 years recommend consuming no more than one meal of fresh swordfish, shark or tuna steak each month. A recent study revealed that PCBs and other toxins in farmed salmon are significantly higher than in the wild species. Although the levels of PCBs are well below recommended limits, for now it is advisable to choose wild salmon whenever possible. The benefits of fish consumption (including tinned tuna) far outweigh the risks, and a healthy diet should contain 3 servings of fish per week.

CRISPY TUNA BALLS

The following recipe is designed to be made in bulk and frozen. Individual portions are then defrosted and baked.

1 medium potato, baked

1 egg, beaten

1 tin white tuna (water-packed), drained

1 tbsp red onion, finely diced

2 cups cornflakes

1 tbsp olive oil

• Cut potato in half and scoop out the inside. In blender or food processor, mix potato, egg, tuna and onion.

• Pour cornflakes into plastic bag. Using rolling pin, crush cornflakes until they are the consistency of bread crumbs.

• Scoop 1 tbsp of tuna mince and form into ball. Place ball in bag and shake until thoroughly coated with cornflakes mixture.

• Place tuna balls in airtight freezer bags and freeze.

• *To serve:* Defrost tuna balls. Spread oil on baking sheet. Place tuna balls on sheet and bake in 350°F oven for 10 minutes. Flip and bake for another 10 minutes. When cooked, tuna balls should be crispy and golden in color.

Yield: 16 to 18 balls

CRISPY B.C. SALMON BALLS

The following recipe is designed to be made in bulk and frozen. Individual portions are then defrosted and baked.

1 medium potato, baked

1 egg, beaten

10 oz salmon, skin and bones
    removed, cut in cubes

1 tsp chopped fresh dill (optional)

Dash lemon juice

1 tbsp onion, finely diced

2 cups cornflakes, crushed

2 tbsp olive oil

• Scoop out the inside of the potato. In blender or food processor, purée egg, salmon, dill (if using), lemon juice and onion.

• Pour cornflakes into plastic bag. Use rolling pin to crush cornflakes until they are the consistency of bread crumbs.

• Scoop 1 tbsp of salmon mince and form into ball. Place ball in bag and shake until thoroughly coated with cornflakes mixture.

• Place salmon balls in freezer bags and freeze.

• *To serve:* Defrost individual portion. Spread oil on baking sheet. Place salmon balls on sheet and bake in 350°F oven for 10 minutes. Flip and bake for another 10 minutes. When done, salmon balls should be crispy and golden brown.

Yield: 16 to 18 balls

FRITTATA

2 potatoes, washed, peeled and
    cut in cubes
I tbsp salt-free butter
10 eggs, beaten

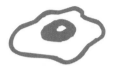

WHAT ARE
OMEGA-3 EGGS?

As little as 2 to 3 servings of fish
per week is thought to reduce the
risk of heart disease and stroke in
adults, and, when included in the
maternal diet, it can enhance newborn brain and retinal development. Recently, omega-3 eggs
have been developed that contain
300 to 500 times more omega-3
than regular eggs. Researchers
fed hens a diet of marine algae,
also the source of omega-3 for
the marine food chain and the
explanation as to the high quantity
of omega-3 in fish. Consuming
one omega-3 egg is equivalent to
consuming one serving of fish.

• In pan of boiling water, par-
boil potatoes for 5 to 10 minutes, just until tender but not
cooked through.
• In frying pan, heat butter
over medium heat and sauté
potatoes for 10 minutes.
• Combine potatoes and eggs,
mixing thoroughly. Pour mixture into greased 8 x 8 baking
dish. Bake in 400°F oven for
about 20 minutes, or until frit-
tata is golden brown around
the edges and just firm to
touch. If in doubt, insert a
knife into the middle; it should
come out clean.

Yield: Fills one 8 x 8-inch pan

PIZZA SOLDIERS

I slice whole-wheat bread

I tsp tomato paste

1/4 cup grated mozzarella cheese
(I oz)

THE SCRAMBLER

I tbsp salt-free butter

4 eggs

1/3 cup grated Cheddar cheese
(1.5 oz)

I tomato, skinned and diced
(recipe, page 60)

I tbsp chopped fresh basil
(optional)

• Lightly toast bread.

• Thinly spread tomato paste on toast and top with cheese.

• Broil about 2 minutes or until cheese melts.

• Remove crust and cut in strips.

Yield: 1 serving

• In frying pan, melt butter.

• In bowl, thoroughly whisk eggs and cheese together and add mixture to pan. Scramble eggs over low heat until cooked.

• Remove from heat. Add tomato and basil (if using); stir until combined.

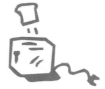

Yield: 2 servings

POTATO WEDGES

These potato wedges, a healthy alternative to store-bought french fries, are perfect for little hands to grasp. Serve alone, or with either homemade Tomato Sauce (recipe, page 61) or your baby's favorite purée.

I baking potato, scrubbed, blemishes removed

2 tbsp olive oil

• Cut potato in half lengthwise. Segment each half into 5 to 6 sections, depending on the size of the potato.
• In bowl, toss segments with olive oil. Roast in 375°F oven for 30 minutes. Flip and roast until potatoes are golden brown, 20 to 30 minutes more.

Yield: 10 to 12 potato wedges

CHILDHOOD OBESITY

Childhood obesity is increasing at an alarming rate, due to a greater reliance on and availability of convenience food and a more sedentary lifestyle. There is also a known hereditary component to obesity. Although it is unnecessary and unhealthy to restrict fats for babies under 2 years old, your doctor may address fat intake by the time your child turns 2 years old, if she exceeds upper weight limits on standardized growth curves (see Appendix III). Your doctor may advise reducing the fat content of milk by switching from whole-fat milk (3.25% m.f.) to reduced-fat milk (I% or 2% m.f.) after the second birthday. It is a good practice with all babies and children to avoid using food as a comfort for disappointment or pain, or using fast food or sweets as a reward. After all, obesity and its health consequences are no treat.

CHICKEN POTPIE

2 tbsp olive oil

1/2 onion, diced

2 stalks celery, washed, trimmed
and diced

I tbsp chopped fresh tarragon
(optional)

I0 mushrooms, thinly sliced

I lb minced chicken

I 1/2 cups low-sodium or Salt-Free
Chicken Stock (recipe, page
66)

2 carrots, washed, peeled and
cut in bite-size pieces

I cup broccoli florets, washed

I tbsp chopped fresh parsley
(optional)

4 large potatoes, washed, peeled
and chopped

1/2 cup (3.25%) milk

4 tbsp salt-free butter

• In large frying pan heat 1 tbsp oil over medium heat and sauté onion, celery and tarragon (if using) for 5 minutes. Add remaining tbsp of oil, and mushrooms; continue to sauté, stirring occasionally, for 15 minutes. Stir in minced chicken; continue to sauté for 10 minutes.

• Add chicken stock, carrots and broccoli; bring to a boil. Reduce heat and simmer until vegetables are tender, stirring occasionally.

• Remove from heat. Add parsley (if using); stir.

• In pot of salted, boiling water, cook potato for topping until tender. Drain well; mash with milk and butter. Spread a layer of chicken mixture in each airtight container. Top with potato. Freeze.

• *To serve:* Defrost in refrigerator. Bake in 350°F oven until pie is bubbling around the edges. Dotting pie with butter and broiling for last 2 minutes of cooking time will make the topping golden brown and crispy.

Yield: 5 to 6 small containers

SHEPHERD'S PIE

1 tbsp olive oil

1/2 onion, diced

1 stalk celery, washed, trimmed
and diced

1 lb ground beef

1 carrot, washed, peeled and cut
in bite-size pieces

1 cup canned whole-kernel corn,
rinsed and drained

1 can (14 oz) diced tomatoes

4 tbsp tomato paste

1 tbsp chopped fresh parsley,
(optional)

4 large potatoes

1/2 cup (3.25%) milk

4 tbsp salt-free butter

• In frying pan, heat oil; sauté onion and celery on low heat until onion is translucent, about 5 minutes. Add beef and continue to sauté until it is no longer pink, about 10 minutes.

• Add carrot, corn, tomatoes, tomato paste and parsley (if using); mix thoroughly. Simmer, partially covered, until carrots are tender, about 25 minutes.

• In a pot of boiling, salted water cook the potato until tender; drain well. Mash with milk and butter. Layer meat in small airtight containers; top with potato. Freeze.

• *To serve:* Defrost and bake in 350°F oven until pie is bubbling around the edges. Dotting pie with butter and broiling for last 2 minutes of cooking time will make the topping golden brown and crispy.

Yield: 5 to 6 small containers

FISH PIE

I lb halibut or other white fish,
   skin and bones removed
2 1/2 cups (3.25%) milk
I bay leaf
2 carrots, peeled and cut in
   bite-size pieces
I tbsp butter
I tbsp flour (approx)
I 1/2 cups grated Cheddar cheese,
   firmly packed (6 oz)
4 hard-boiled eggs, crumbled
I tbsp chopped fresh chives
   (optional)
4 large potatoes
4 tbsp salt-free butter

• Cut fish into cubes. Place in saucepan with bay leaf; cover with 2 cups of milk. Bring to a light boil; reduce heat and simmer until fish flakes, about 20 minutes. Drain fish; set poaching milk aside. Once cool, crumble fish in bowl with fingers, checking for bones.
• In steamer, cook carrots over boiling water until tender.
• In large saucepan, whisk together butter and flour over medium heat until paste forms. Slowly add 1/2 cup of poaching milk, whisking until lumps disappear. Add both cheese and another 1/2 cup of poaching milk, whisking until cheese melts and sauce thickens.
• Once sauce is smooth and creamy, add to fish. Mix in carrots, eggs and chives (if using).
• In pot of salted, boiling water, cook potatoes until tender. Drain well; mash with the remaining 1/2 cup milk and butter.
• Layer fish mixture in airtight container. Top with potato. Freeze.
• *To serve:* Defrost. Bake in 350°F until pie is bubbling at the edges, 20 to 25 minutes. Dotting pie with butter and broiling for last 2 minutes of cooking time will make the topping golden brown and crispy.

Yield: 4 to 5 small containers

PIZZA

This easy-to-make pizza is a crowd-pleaser among children of all ages. It can be made with a variety of toppings, and kids love the opportunity to make their own. Let them experiment!

I 10-inch soft flour tortilla
I tbsp tomato paste
1/3 cup grated Cheddar cheese
   (1.5 oz)
I slice Black Forest ham, cut in
   strips

• Broil tortilla in oven until edges begin to turn golden brown, 4 to 5 minutes.
• Allow tortilla to cool; spread evenly with tomato paste. Sprinkle with cheese and ham.
• Broil in oven until cheese melts, 1 to 2 minutes.
• Allow to cool. Using scissors, cut in wedges and serve.

Yield: 1 serving

BAKED MACARONI AND CHEESE

Make the following recipe in a baking dish and serve as a meal for the entire family. For smaller babies, individual portions can be pulsed in the blender or food processor until desired consistency is reached. Leftovers can be stored in the fridge, making convenient baby and toddler meals. Alternatively, pour the pasta and sauce mixture into airtight containers and freeze. *To serve:* Defrost. Warm by baking in 350°F oven or simmering over low heat in a saucepan.

2 tbsp flour
2 tbsp salt-free butter
2 cups (3.25%) milk
4 cups macaroni
3 cups grated sharp Cheddar
   cheese, firmly packed (I lb)
I cup grated Parmesan cheese
   (4 oz)
2 tbsp salt-free butter
4 tbsp whole-wheat bread
   crumbs

FRUIT SHAKE

The following shakes can be made with fresh fruit, but frozen berries give them a refreshing frostiness.

I cup (3.25%) milk

I banana

1/2 cup high-fat (over 3%) plain
   yogurt

1/2 cup frozen mixed berries

• In blender, purée milk, banana, yogurt and berries until shake is frothy.

Yield: 4 servings

VERY BERRY SHAKE

I cup orange juice

I banana

1/2 cup frozen mixed berries

• In blender, purée orange juice, banana and berries until shake is frothy.

Yield: 2 servings

• *To make cheese sauce:* In saucepan, whisk together 2 tbsp of butter and flour over medium heat. Add 1 cup of milk; continue to whisk until lumps disappear. Add Cheddar cheese and remainder of milk, whisking until cheese melts. Stir in 1/2 cup of Parmesan cheese; allow sauce to thicken.

• Cook macaroni al dente. Mix with cheese sauce until pasta is thoroughly coated.

• Pour mixture into greased medium-size baking dish.

• In saucepan, melt 2 tbsp of butter. Add bread crumbs; stir until bread crumbs are coated. Remove from heat; mix with remaining Parmesan cheese. Sprinkle bread crumbs over macaroni and cheese.

• Bake in 350°F oven until warm (approx 30 minutes).

Yield: 1 medium-size baking dish

SILLY SANDWICH IDEAS

Use cookie cutters to produce an entertaining variety of sandwich shapes and sizes. And sandwiches cut with cookie rounds can be decorated with such extras as sliced cherry tomatoes and soft-cooked carrots to become funny faces. Mixing cream cheese with one of your baby's top purées makes a tasty sandwich filling; cream cheese mixed with apple purée, mashed avocado or mashed banana are just a few possibilities. Remember to make your sandwiches with whole-wheat bread. This is your chance to form life-long habits.

DIPS

Even fussy eaters enjoy dips. The following easy-to-prepare dips make savory, nutritious snacks that can be enjoyed by the whole family. Instead of serving them with chips, try whole-wheat toast strips, whole-grain crackers or steamed vegetables.

HUMMUS

I can (19 oz) chick-peas, drained
   and rinsed
I tbsp olive oil
I tbsp fresh lemon juice

• In blender or food processor, purée chick-peas, oil and lemon juice.
• Serve with toasted whole-wheat pita bread or steamed vegetables.

GUACAMOLE

I ripe avocado, washed
I tbsp high-fat (over 3%) yogurt
Dash lemon juice

• Cut avocado in half; remove pit and scoop out fruit.
• In small bowl, mash avocado with a fork. Add yogurt and lemon juice. Mix thoroughly.
• Serve with steamed vegetables or whole-wheat toast strips.

ROASTED RED PEPPER HUMMUS

I sweet red pepper, washed
I can (19 oz) chick-peas, drained
   and rinsed
1/3 cup high-fat (over 3%) plain
   yogurt
I clove garlic, crushed
I tbsp chopped fresh basil
   (optional)

• *To roast a pepper:* Place pepper on a large sheet of tinfoil; broil in oven, 10 to 15 minutes. Watching carefully, rotate the pepper as it begins to bubble and darken. Once the entire skin has bubbled, remove from oven; wrap in foil. Allow pepper to sit for 20 minutes (to enable it to continue to cook). Once pepper is cool, peel away skin; remove seeds and stem.
• In blender or food processor, purée pepper, chick-peas, yogurt and garlic until smooth.
• Pour dip into a bowl; sprinkle with basil (if using).
• Serve with steamed vegetables and toasted whole-wheat pita triangles.

JACKET POTATOES

Baked potatoes are a good source of both vitamin C and carbo-hydrates. Use a microwave to bake the potato and you'll find the following recipes quick and easy to prepare. Don't forget to prick the potato with a fork several times before microwaving. Cooking times will vary, so refer to your manufacturer's instructions.

VEGETABLE RAGOUT POTATO

I potato, baked

I/3 cup Vegetable Ragout (recipe,
  page 134)

I/3 cup grated Cheddar cheese
  (1.5 oz)

5 thin slices green onion

I tbsp chopped fresh basil
  (optional)

• Split potato in half and open. Pour vegetable ragout over potato; sprinkle with cheese.
• Bake in 350°F oven until cheese melts and mixture is warmed through, 10 to 15 minutes. Remove from oven. Sprinkle with onion and basil (if using). Serve.

Yield: 1 serving

CHEESY POTATO DELUXE

I potato, baked

I/3 cup high-fat (over 3%) plain
  yogurt

2 tbsp grated Parmesan cheese

I/2 cup grated Cheddar cheese
  (2 oz)

5 thin slices green onion (optional)

• Cut potato in half; scoop out flesh, leaving enough around the sides so that the potato keeps its shape.
• In bowl, mash potato; mix with yogurt and cheeses. Scoop the mixture back into the potato. Bake in 350°F oven until mixture is warmed through, 10 to 15 minutes. Broil for 2 minutes to make the topping crispy. Sprinkle with green onion. Serve.

Yield: 1 serving

CHEESY BROCCOLI POTATO

I potato, baked

3 broccoli florets, washed, steamed and diced

2 tbsp high-fat (over 3%) plain yogurt

1/3 cup grated Cheddar cheese (1.5 oz)

5 thin slices green onion

• Cut potato in half. Scoop out flesh, leaving enough around the sides so that the potato keeps its shape.

• Mash potato; mix with broccoli, yogurt and cheese. Scoop the mixture back into the potato. Bake in 350°F oven until warmed through, 10 to 15 minutes. Broil for last 2 minutes to make the topping crispy. Sprinkle with green onion. Serve.

Yield: 1 serving

SOUPS

Many toddlers who refuse to eat vegetables will happily eat them disguised in soup. The following recipes can be served to the whole family. All require either low-sodium or salt-free chicken stock. Low-sodium chicken stock is now conveniently available in most grocery stores, or you can make your own Salt-Free Chicken Stock (recipe, page 66).

LENTIL SOUP

2 tbsp olive oil

I onion, diced

I stalk celery, washed, trimmed
　　and diced

2 cloves garlic, crushed

I tsp curry powder

I tbsp cumin

4 carrots, washed, peeled and
　　sliced

2 large potatoes, washed, peeled
　　and cubed

I0 cups low-sodium or Salt-Free
　　Chicken Stock (recipe, page 66)

I can (I4 oz) diced tomatoes

I I/3 cups dried green lentils,
　　rinsed and drained

I/4 cup chopped fresh cilantro
　　(optional)

• In large pot, heat oil; sauté onion, celery, garlic, curry powder and cumin over medium heat for 10 minutes. Add carrots, potatoes and stock; bring to a boil. Reduce heat and simmer until vegetables are tender, about 20 minutes.

• Using strainer, separate stock from vegetables; set stock aside.

• In blender or food processor, purée vegetables to a fine consistency.

• Return mixture to pot; over low heat mix vegetables and stock together. Add tomatoes and lentils; bring to a boil. Reduce heat and simmer, partially covered, for 1 hour.

• Remove from heat; mix in cilantro (if using). Allow to cool.

• Pour into airtight containers. Freeze.

MOROCCAN VEGETABLE SOUP

3 tbsp olive oil

I onion, diced

I stalk celery, washed, trimmed
and diced

I can (19 oz) chick-peas, rinsed
and drained

I tbsp cumin (approx)

I clove garlic, crushed

10 cups low-sodium chicken stock
or Salt-Free Chicken Stock
(recipe, page 66)

I potato, washed, peeled and
cubed

I cup broccoli florets, washed

4 carrots, washed, peeled and
sliced

I can (14 oz) diced tomatoes

2 large handfuls spinach, washed
and trimmed

• In large pot, sauté onion and celery in oil over medium heat until onion is translucent, about 5 minutes.

• Add chick-peas, cumin and garlic; continue to sauté for another 10 minutes.

• Add chicken stock, potato, broccoli, carrots and tomatoes. Bring to a rapid boil, reduce heat and simmer, partially covered, for 1 hour; stir occasionally. Add spinach for the last 5 minutes of cooking time.

• Pour mixture through a strainer, separating stock from vegetables; set stock aside.

• In blender or food processor, purée vegetables to a rough consistency. In pot over medium heat, mix vegetables and stock.

• Allow to cool. Pour contents into airtight containers and freeze.

VEGETABLE BARLEY
SOUP

3 tbsp olive oil

I onion, diced

3 stalks celery, washed, trimmed
and sliced

2 cloves garlic, crushed

10 cups low-sodium or Salt-Free
Chicken Stalk (recipe, page 66)

I can (14 oz) diced tomatoes

1/2 cup barley, rinsed and drained

3 carrots, washed, peeled and
sliced

I potato, washed, peeled and cut
in bite-size pieces

1/4 cup chopped fresh parsley
(optional)

• In large pot, heat oil over medium heat; sauté onion, celery and garlic for 10 minutes.

• Add chicken stock, tomatoes and barley, and bring to a boil. Reduce and simmer for 30 minutes, partially covered. Stir occasionally.

• Add carrots, potato and parsley (if using). Continue to simmer until vegetables are tender, about 30 minutes.

• Allow soup to cool. Pour into airtight containers. Freeze.

• *Tip:* For younger toddlers you may choose to use a blender or food processor to purée before freezing.

BROCCOLI SOUP

This hearty soup can also be served with grated Parmesan cheese: simply stir 2 tbsp of grated cheese into a bowl of soup, and serve.

3 tbsp olive oil

I onion, diced

8 cups low-sodium or Salt-Free
    Chicken Stock (recipe, page 66)

2 medium bunches broccoli,
    washed and cut in florets

I potato, washed, peeled and cut
    in cubes

• In large pot, heat oil over medium heat; sauté onion until translucent, anout 5 minutes. Add chicken stock and vegetables. Bring to rapid boil, reduce heat and simmer until vegetables are tender, about 20 to 25 minutes.

• Using strainer, separate vegetables from stock; set stock aside.

• In blender or food processor, purée vegetables to a rough consistency.

• In pot over low heat, combine puréed vegetables and stock; mix.

• Allow soup to cool. Pour into airtight containers. Freeze.

Appendix I: Resources

American Academy of Allergy, Asthma & Immunology
555 East Wells Street
Suite 1100
Milwaukee, WI 53202-3823
Tel: (414) 272-6071
Patient Information and Physician Referral Line:
(800) 822-2762 (toll-free)
www.aaaai.org

National Asthma Council, Australia
Asthma Management Handbook 2002 (online)
www.nationalasthma.org.au

CANADIAN DENTAL ASSOCIATION
1815 Alta Vista Dr.
Ottawa, ON K1G 3Y6
Tel: (613) 523-1770 or (800) 267-6354 (toll-free)
www.cda-adc.ca

CANADIAN PAEDIATRIC SOCIETY
2305 St. Laurent Blvd.
Ottawa ON K1G 4J8
Tel: (613) 526-9397
www.cps.ca/english/index.htm

DIETITIANS OF CANADA
480 University Ave., Suite 604
Toronto, ON M5G 1V2
Tel: (416) 596-0857
www.dietitians.ca

GLUTEN INTOLERANCE/COELIAC DISEASE SUPPORT
Coeliac UK
Suites A–D, Octagon Court
High Wycombe
Bucks HP11 2HS
United Kingdom
www.coeliac.co.uk

THE COELIAC SOCIETY OF AUSTRALIA
306 Victoria Avenue, First Floor
Chatswood NSW 2067
Tel: 61-2-941-4100
www.coeliac.org.au

HEALTH CANADA
Address Locator 0900C2
Ottawa, ON K1A 0K9
Tel: (613) 957-2991 or (800) 225-0709 (toll-free)
TTY: (800) 267-1245
www.hc-sc.gc.ca

HEALTHY EATING
Recommended DVD:
Yummy in My Tummy: Good Eating Habits for Life
To order:
www.liandrea.com

IMMUNIZATION
Recommended book:
Your Child's Best Shot: A Parent's Guide to Vaccination, by Ronald
Gold, MD, MPH
Published by the Canadian Paediatric Society:
www.cps.ca/english/publications/Bookstore

IRON-DEFICIENCY ANEMIA
Anemia Institute—National Office
151 Bloor St. W., Suite 600
Toronto, ON M5S 1S4
Tel: (416) 969-7431
www.anemiainstitute.org

LA LECHE LEAGUE
The La Leche League website provides a list of contacts for countries
around the world. Information on lactose intolerance is also available.
www.lalecheleague.org

THE NATIONAL INSTITUTE OF HEALTH / NATIONAL INSTITUTE OF DIGESTIVE DISEASES (U.S.)
For information on lactose intolerance.
http://digestive.niddk.nih.gov/ddiseases/pubs/lactoseintolerance/

AMERICAN ACADEMY OF PEDIATRICS
www.aap.org
Resource Books (Click on Bookstore & Publications):
Caring for Your Baby and Young Child, Birth to Age 5
Guide to Your Child's Allergies and Asthma
Guide to Your Child's Nutrition
Guide to Your Child's Sleep
Guide to Your Child's Symptoms
Your Baby's First Year

ST. JOHN AMBULANCE
National Office
1900 City Park Drive, Suite 400
Ottawa, ON K1A 1A3
Tel: (613) 236-7461
www.sja.ca

Appendix II:
Growth Charts

The following are growth charts from the U.S. Center of Disease Control. The charts are based on large population studies and are independent of race and ethnicity. They also include both breast-fed and formula-fed infants. To plot your baby's progress, choose either the male or female chart and find the age in months on the horizontal access and trace up to the height or weight on the vertical access. The point plotted corresponds to a "growth percentile." For example, a male baby found to be in the 75% range for height is taller than 75% of all male babies his age and shorter than 25% of all male babies his age. Growth generally follows along a percentile curve throughout infancy. Concerns arise when growth is below or above expected percentiles or when growth deviates from predicted patterns.

Birth to 36 months: Boys
Length-for-age and Weight-for-age percentiles

NAME _____

RECORD # _____

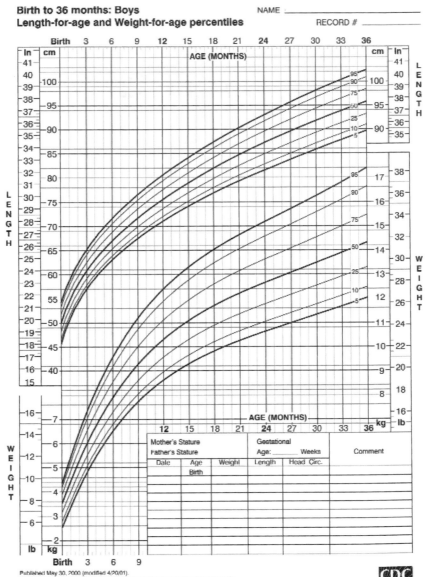

AGE (MONTHS)

LENGTH

WEIGHT

Mother's Stature			Gestational		Comment
Father's Stature			Age: _____ Weeks		
Date	Age	Weight	Length	Head Circ.	
	Birth				

Published May 30, 2000 (modified 4/20/01).
SOURCE: Developed by the National Center for Health Statistics in collaboration with
the National Center for Chronic Disease Prevention and Health Promotion (2000).
http://www.cdc.gov/growthcharts

SAFER • HEALTHIER • PEOPLE™

Birth to 36 months: Girls
Length-for-age and Weight-for-age percentiles

NAME _____

RECORD # _____

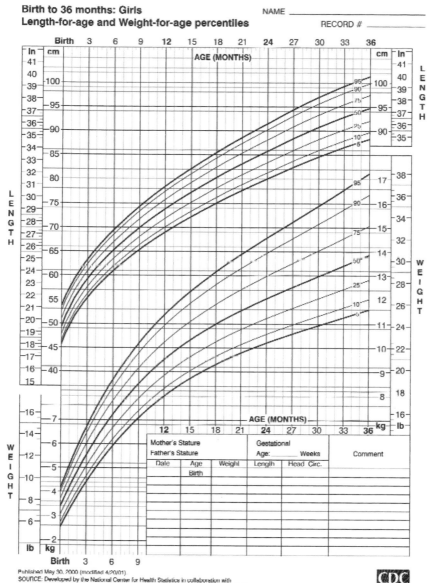

Published May 30, 2000 (modified 4/20/01).
SOURCE: Developed by the National Center for Health Statistics in collaboration with
the National Center for Chronic Disease Prevention and Health Promotion (2000).
http://www.cdc.gov/growthcharts

CDC
SAFER·HEALTHIER·PEOPLE™

163

Appendix III: References

1. Canadian Paediatric Society, Dietitians of Canada and Health Canada. Nutrition for Healthy Term Infants. Ottawa: Minister of Public Works and Government Services; 1998.

2. Health Canada. Exclusive Breastfeeding Duration: 2004. Health Canada Recommendations, 2004.

3. American Academy of Pediatrics Work Group on Breastfeeding Policy Statement. Breastfeeding and the use of human milk (RE9729). *Pediatrics.* 1997;100:1035–1039.

4. Beaudry M et al. Relationship between infant feeding and infections during the first six months of life. *J. Pediatr.* 1995; 126:191–197.

5. Ford RPK, Taylor BJ, Mitchell EA. Breastfeeding and the risk of sudden infant death syndrome. *Int J Epidemiol.* 1993;22:885–890.

6. Horwood LJ and Ferguson DM. Breastfeeding and later cognitive development and academic outcomes. *Pediatrics.* 1998;101:9.

7. Temboury et al. Influence of breastfeeding on the infant's intellectual development. *J. Pediatr Gastroenter Nutr.* 1994;18:32–36.

8. Chandra RK. Five year follow-up of high risk infants with family history of allergy who were exclusively breast-fed or fed partial whey hydrosylate,

soy, and conventional cow's milk formulas. *J Pediatr Gastroenterol Nutr.* 1997;24:380–388.

9. Saarinen UM, Kajosaari M. Breastfeeding as prophylaxis against atopic disease: prospective follow-up study until 17 years old. *Lancet.* 1995;346:1065–1069.

10. Greene-Finestone L, Feldman W, Heick H, et al. Prevalence and risk factors of iron depletion and iron deficiency anaemia among infants in Ottawa-Carlton. *Can Diet Assoc J.* 1991;52:20–23.

11. Pizarro F, Yip R, Dallman PR, et al. Iron status with different infant feeding regimens: relevance to screening and prevention of iron deficiency. *J Pediatr.* 1991;118:687–692.

12. Cumming RG, Klineberg RJ. Breastfeeding and other reproductive factors and the risk of hip fractures in elderly women. *Int J Epidemiol.* 1993;22:684–691.

13. Melton LJ et al. Influence of breastfeeding and other reproductive factors on bone mass later in life. *Osteopros Int.* 1993;3:76–83.

14. Newcomb PA et al. Lactation and reduced risk of premenopausal breast cancer. *N Engl J Med.* 1994;330:81–87.

15. Rosenblatt KA, Thomas DB. WHO collaborative study of neoplasia and steroid contraceptives. *Int J Epidemiol.* 1993;22:192–197.

16. Dewey et al. Maternal weight-loss patterns during prolonged lactation. *Am J Clin Nutr.* 1993;58:162–166.

17. Canadian Paediatric Society, Indian and Inuit Health Committee. Vitamin D supplementation for northern native communities. *Can Med Assoc J.* 1988;138:229–230.

18. Lawrence et al. Prevention of rickets and vitamin D deficiency. New guidelines for vitamin D intake. *Pediatrics.* 2003;111:908–910.

19. Health Canada. Vitamin D Supplementation for Breastfed Infants: 2004. Health Canada Recommendations, 2004.

20. Lawton ME. Alcohol in breastmilk. *Aust N Z J Obstet Gynaecol.* 1985;25:71–73.

21. Little RE et al. Maternal alcohol use during breast-feeding and infant mental and motor development at one year. *New Engl J Med.* 1989;7:425–430.

22. Menella JA, Gerrish CJ. Effects of exposure to alcohol in mother's milk on infant sleep. *Pediatrics.* 1998;101(5):2.

23. Canadian Institute of Child Health. National breastfeeding guidelines for health care providers. 2nd ed., Ottawa; 1996.

24. Smith MM, Lifshitz F. Excess fruit juice consumption as a contributing factor in nonorganic failure to thrive. *Pediatrics.* 1994;93:438–443.

25. Canadian Paediatric Society, Nutrition Committee. The use of fluoride in infants and children. *Paediatrics & Child Health.* 2002;7(8):569–572. Reference no. N02-01.

26. Lucassen et al. Effectiveness of treatments for infantile colic: systematic review. *BMJ.* 1998;316:1563–1569.

27. The American Academy of Pediatrics. *Guide to Your Child's Nutrition.* New York: Random House, 1999.

28. Bock, SA. The natural history of adverse reactions to foods. *Allergy Proceedings.* 1986;7:504–510.

29. Canadian Paediatric Society. Fatal anaphylactic reactions to food in children. *Can Med Assoc J.* 1994;150:337–339.

30. Bock SA, Atkins F. Patterns of food hypersensitivity during sixteen years of double-blind placebo controlled food challenges. *J. Pediatr.* 1990;117:561–567.

31. Dewey et al. Breastfed infants are leaner than formula fed infants at one year of age: The Darling Study. *Am J Clin Nutr.* 1993;57:140–145.

32. Canadian Paediatric Society and Health Canada. Report of the Joint Working Group. Nutrition Recommendations Update: Dietary Fat and Children. Ottawa. 1994.

33. Pickering et al. Modulation of the immune system by human milk and infant formula containing nucleotides. *Paediatrics.* 1998;101:242–249.

34. Schutze GE et al. The home environment and salmonellosis in children. *Pediatrics*. 1999;103:1.

35. Canadian Paediatric Society. Meeting the needs of infants and young children: an update. *Can Med Assoc J*. 1991;144:1451–1454.

36. Feldman W, Randel P. Screening children for lead exposure in Canada. In: Canadian Task Force on the Periodic Health Examination. *Canadian Guide to Clinical Preventative Health Care*. Ottawa: Health Canada; 1994;268–288.

37. Canadian Paediatric Society. Effective discipline for children. *Paediatrics & Child Health*. 1997;2(1):29–33.

38. Hodge et al. Consumption of oily fish and childhood asthma risk. *MJA*. 1996;164:137–140.

39. Stevens et al. Omega-3 fatty acids and boys with behaviour, learning and health problems. *Physiology and Behaviour*. 1996;59:915–920.

40. American Academy of Pediatrics Provisional Committee on Quality Improvement, Subcommittee on Acute Gastroenteritis. Practice parameter: the management of acute gastroenteritis in young children. *Pediatrics*. 1996;97:424–435.

41. Canadian Paediatric Society, Nutrition Committee. Oral rehydration therapy and early refeeding in the management of gastroenteritis. *Can J Paediatr*. 1994b;1:160–164.

42. Yagev Y, Koren G. Eating fish during pregnancy, risk of exposure to toxic levels of methylmercury. *Canadian Family Physician*. 2002;48:1619–1621.

43. Vallejo F et al. Phenolic compound contents in edible parts of broccoli inflorescences after domestic cooking. *Journal of the Science of Food and Agriculture*. 2003;83:1511–1516.

44. Hites et al. Global assessment of organic contaminants in farmed salmon. *Science* 2004;303:226–229.

45. Craig-Schmidt MC. Isomeric fatty acids: evaluating status and implications for maternal and child health. *Lipids*. 2001;36:997–1006.

Recipe Index

Halibut Fish Sticks, 136
Hash, Easy Beef, 79
Hummus, 149

Okanagan Summer Chicken, 105
Okanagan Summer Salad, 58

I J K

L

M

General Index

ADHD (attention deficit hyperactivity disorder), 118
Alcohol, 11
Allergies
  and breastfeeding, 6
  common food, 26
  to cow's milk, 13, 26, 27
  diagnosis of food, 26
  to eggs, 27
  family history of food, 6, 26–27
  and introduction of solid food, 22–23, 25
  management of food, 27–28
  to peanuts, 26, 59
  prevalence of food, 25
  severe food, 26
  to soy, 13, 26, 27
  to wheat, 23, 26, 27–28, 71, 99
Anaphylaxis, 26
Anemia. See Iron-deficiency anemia
Antioxidants, 36, 60
Appetite, 102
  poor or decreased, 76, 103, 124
  of toddlers, 113, 131, 132
  and zinc in diet, 99
Apple juice, unpasteurized, 66
Asthma, 6, 115
Attention deficit hyperactivity disorder (ADHD), 118

Baby food. See Solid food
Beans, 96

Beta-carotene, 36
Blood in stool, 58, 66, 124
Bone development, 9, 28, 44, 87
Bottle
  self-feeding with, 75
  sterilization of, 14
  switching to cup from, 75
  used as pacifier, 75
Bowel diseases, reducing
  risk of, 6
Bowel movements
  change in normal pattern of, 58, 62
  at 1 week of age, 9
Brain development, 6, 12, 33, 46, 47, 116, 122, 140
Breads, introduction of, 126
Breast milk
  alcohol in, 11
  composition of, 8
  expressing and storing, 10
  fatty acids in, 12, 17
  iron in, 10
  taurine in, 13
  warming bags or bottles of, 11, 14
Breastfeeding
  alcohol consumption while, 11
  benefits of, 6–7, 12, 13, 17
  frequency of, 9
  getting started, 8–9
  health conditions that may preclude, 11

ACKNOWLEDGMENTS

We would like to thank a number of people without whose help and support this book would not be what it is today: Dr. Cheryl Mutch, Dr. Yvonne Ou, Dr. RuLin Fuong, Anne Lindsay, Karen Fryer, Val Bradshaw, Elaine Donaldson and Random House Canada.

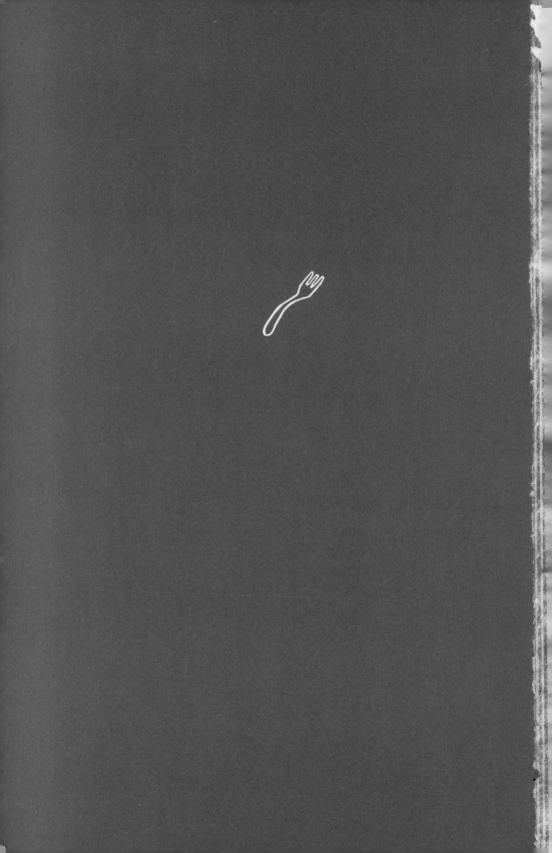